Depression
and Your Child

Depression and Your Child

A Guide for Parents and Caregivers

DEBORAH SERANI

ROWMAN & LITTLEFIELD
Lanham • Boulder • New York • London

Published by Rowman & Littlefield
4501 Forbes Boulevard, Suite 200, Lanham, Maryland 20706
www.rowman.com

Unit A, Whitacre Mews, 26-34 Stannary Street, London SE11 4AB

British Library Cataloguing in Publication Information Available

Library of Congress Cataloging-in-Publication Data

The hardback edition of this book was previously cataloged by the Library of Congress as follows:

Serani, Deborah, 1961–
  Depression and your child : a guide for parents and caregivers / Deborah Serani.
    pages cm
  Includes bibliographical references and index.
  1. Depression in children—Popular works. 2. Depression in adolescence—Popular works. 3. Parenting. I. Title.
  RJ506.D4S46 2013
  618.92'8527—dc23   2013014858

ISBN: 978-1-4422-2145-1 (cloth : alk. paper)
ISBN: 978-1-4422-4446-7 (pbk. : alk. paper)
ISBN: 978-1-4422-2146-8 (electronic)

∞™ The paper used in this publication meets the minimum requirements of American National Standard for Information Sciences—Permanence of Paper for Printed Library Materials, ANSI/NISO Z39.48-1992.

Printed in the United States of America

For my parents, Carmela and Silvio

Contents

Acknowledgments

To write is to work in solitude, in isolation. And I love that process. To be published requires working alongside others, and I love that process, too. To Senior Editor Suzanne Staszak-Silva, I thank you for your discerning editorial eye, your compassionate listening, and your gentle manner. You made my work shine more brilliantly than I could have ever imagined. To my publicist, Sam Caggiula, your enthusiasm and support were like a faraway beacon, giving me hope when I struggled uphill in my writing journey. I'm also grateful to Patricia Stevenson, production editor, for bringing my book to life; to Desiree Reid for your beautiful copyedit; and to the marketing and sales teams at Rowman & Littlefield. Many thanks to my colleagues who offered notes and insights, and those I've worked with who allowed their stories to be told. To my home-base team, Ira and Rebecca, thank you for letting me fly away for hours on end to write—and, finally, to my sisters and parents for loving me through all the ups and downs and in-betweens life has thrown my way.

Introduction

When you held your child for the very first time, you were likely brimming with pride and joy. Your heart swelling with enormous love, you're swept away with streams of thoughts for what your child needs in this immediate moment—as well as plans and dreams for the future. You expect there to be wondrous adventures your child will experience, as well as bumps in the road along the way. *And that's okay*, you say, because you know that life isn't always an easy journey.

But one thing you probably never considered was how an illness like depression could take hold of your child. And why would you? Up until recently, it was never believed that children could experience depression. Long ago, studies suggested that children and teenagers didn't have the emotional capacity or cognitive development to experience the hopelessness and helplessness of depression.

Today, we know that children, even babies, experience depression. The clinical term is called *pediatric depression*, and rates are higher now than ever before. In the United States alone, evidence suggests that 4 percent of preschool-aged children, 5 percent of school-aged children, and 11 percent of adolescents meet the criteria for major depression.

WHY I WROTE THIS BOOK

Depression and Your Child grew out of my experience of being a clinician who specializes in the treatment of pediatric depression. I wanted to write a parenting book to raise awareness about depressive disorders in children, to teach parents how to find treatment, to offer tips for creating a healthy living environment, and to highlight important adult parenting matters such as self-care, romance, and well-being.

I also wrote this book because I have lived with depression since I was a child. As is the case with pediatric depression, my own depression didn't hit with lightning-like speed. It was more of a slow burn, taking its toll in gnaws and bites before hollowing me out completely. After a suicide attempt as a college sophomore, I found help that finally reduced my depression. Until then, I accepted the sadness, despair, and overwhelming fatigue *as the way my life just was.* I never realized, nor did my parents or any other adults, that I had a clinical disorder. I've since turned the wounds from my childhood into wisdom and believe that sharing the textures of my experiences will help parents realize what their own depressed child is going through.

More than anything else, I want this book to offer hope. As a clinician, proper diagnosis and treatment can be life changing and life saving. As a person living with depression, I have found successful ways to lead a full and meaningful life. I want parents and children who struggle with depression to feel this hope, too—and in these pages, that's what you'll find.

ABOUT THIS BOOK

I'm a teacher at heart. Just about everything I do in my personal and professional life has some aspect of nurturance to it. I want readers to be able to take what's in these pages and apply them to their life. The chapters herein will give you all the necessary requirements needed to parent your child with depression with confidence and success.

You'll learn about the normative patterns and stages of child development, from physical, verbal, cognitive, emotional, and social development. I'll teach you how to observe your child, how to spot potential concerns, and I will give you the insight needed to help diagnose depression. As you read further, I not only outline traditional treatments for pediatric depression but also delve deeply into holistic methods. I'm a great believer that there's more than one way to treat illness—and finding what works for you and your child will be vital. In the pages of this book you'll also find out how to tap school resources for additional support and what kinds of specialists you need to advocate for your depressed child. I discuss the scariest subject matter related to depression—suicide and self-harm—in a manner that is candid and frank, yet hopeful. I want parents to know what to expect from medication if it's needed, from hospitalization if it's necessary, and what kinds of realistic expectations to have regarding what psychotherapy can and can't do when it comes to depression.

A significant emphasis in *Depression and Your Child* is making sure you, as a parent, carve out time for yourself and time for your love life. Chapters include tips for intact families, single parents, and co-parenting arrangements, as well as for caregivers who may need to plan for future caregiving for their depressed child. And because stigma features strongly in the life of anyone who lives with mental illness, a section of myths, facts, and ways to address such stigma is featured. Furthermore, a list of almost four hundred high-profile people, from athletes, actors, and musicians to scientists and world leaders, will help you and your depressed child see that people who have depression can lead meaningful lives.

To broaden the understanding of what's covered in this book, I've included a case study at the end of each chapter. Though the names and other identifying information have been changed to keep confidentiality, reading the stories of these selected cases will help you understand theories, treatments, and techniques.

Finally, worldwide resources to advocacy websites, mental health organizations, parenting associations, suicide hotlines, and pharmacology agencies round out *Depression and Your Child*, making this truly a guidebook for parents.

1

Understanding Child Development

As a young girl, I always felt this looming sense of sadness. I remember feeling tired and sullen a good deal of the time growing up. When I was in school, I was quiet and kept to myself, but these feelings didn't get much better when I was at home. Like Eeyore, the glum little donkey from the Hundred Acre Wood, I was known as a sad sack to friends and family.[1]

Piecing together my interior life along with school reports, my medical history, and my parents' recollections, it's easy to see *now* that I was a depressed child. I was very sensitive, cried easily, was frequently tired and irritable, and was prone to headaches and stomachaches. And then there were the feelings of insecurity that plagued me wherever I went. I never felt good enough or smart enough, strong enough or pretty enough—so I preferred being alone to spending time with friends. I also struggled to concentrate at school, constantly having to work hard to catch up to what was going on in the classroom—as if my focus was moving at a slower pace than everyone else's.

My depressive illness didn't accompany my life as a big, dark cloud shrouding me in blackness. It was a silent partner—hazily clipping the edges of the light, subtly pressing itself against me in ways that made me complacent. Back then, I didn't know I was depressed. I just thought everyone felt and thought the kinds of things I did. And no one—teachers, health professionals, friends, or family—took notice of my depression back then either. This was partly because children weren't thought to experience clinical depression. In addition, my behavioral and emotional presentations weren't extreme, raising flags that I was a kid that needed looking after. I was a good, quiet kid who didn't get into trouble.

But as I got older, my depressive symptoms intensified, challenging me to work harder to shake the negative feelings and physical fatigue. By then, I learned to mask them well by presenting a cheerful exterior publicly while privately feeling sad. I'd force myself to keep social plans with friends and attend extra-help sessions after school to improve my grades, and I even joined sports teams as an antidote to my constant tiredness. Try as I might to fight the dimness of my mood and the distortions of my thoughts, I often ended up canceling on friends, barely passing school subjects, and quitting every sports team before the season ended.

My negative and corrosive thinking made it hard for me to feel hopeful or happy, and soon I descended into a perilous despair. At age nineteen, my junior year of college, a staggering sadness seized, spiraling me into a hopeless frame of mind. Within weeks, I stopped studying, then stopped going to my classes altogether. I remained in bed nearly all day, the depression siphoning out my soul, creating for me a featureless, numbing existence. Soon my judgment clouded, and I lost my sense of thinking clearly. With each passing day, I struggled to keep away thoughts and urges to hurt myself. Unable to control these internal pressures, my emotional collapse led to a plan to die by suicide with a loaded handgun. Luckily, my self-destructive act was interrupted, and I received immediate medical care.

Through the life-saving interventions, I came to learn that as a young girl I'd been living with *dysthymia* and that it had escalated into a *major depressive disorder*. Having both these disorders was called a *double depression*, and it wouldn't be the last time that would challenge me. Some fifteen years later, I found myself in dire straits again, but knowing what risk factors to look for helped save me from plummeting into what could have been another life-threatening situation. I was a trained clinician and realized what was going on. I kept an eye on my mental state just after returning home with my healthy, newborn, beautiful daughter, Rebecca. I started noticing how I was feeling weepy, anxious, and irritable. Thinking it might be the radical hormone changes known as the baby blues, I gave myself some time before checking things out with the doctor. Within months, those symptoms worsened, with negative thoughts, despairing feelings, and self-destructive ideas plaguing me once again. There was no doubt in my mind that I was experiencing another depressive episode—this time it was with the onset of postpartum. I began medication and resumed psychotherapy, and I was feeling better in a matter of weeks.

I have no doubt that if my parents, teachers, coaches, friends, and family knew what to look for back when I was a child, I would've been involved in treatment much earlier in my life. And I strongly believe that earlier intervention would have helped me avoid circling the drain and thinking of suicide. Better late than never, getting treatment in my late teens was life saving and inspirational to me, so much so that I became a student of psychology—and have been an expert psychologist diagnosing and treating depression in children and adults for over twenty years.

Born out of my personal experiences with depression has come my professional need to educate others about how to detect depression, how to treat it, and how to live well in spite of it.

DEFINING NORMAL

Understanding the range of normal development can help determine if your child's thoughts and behaviors warrant concern. First and foremost is the idea of understanding what *normal* is. Many definitions exist, but in my opinion, none get the job done in a single sentence.

There's the intellectual definition: "Normal is conforming to a type, standard, or regular pattern."—*Merriam Webster Dictionary*.[2]

A tongue-in-cheek definition: "Normal is nothing more than a cycle on a washing machine."—Whoopi Goldberg.[3]

And the existential definition: "Nobody realizes that some people expend tremendous energy merely to be normal."—Albert Camus.[4]

Defining normal starts with understanding that each culture has a set of
accepted customs, rituals, traditions, and expectations that guide the population. These agreed-upon norms may be the same from country to country,
they may vary from place to place, or be entirely different from one part of
the world to another. For example, a handshake as a greeting is welcomed
in American, Canadian, and European cultures, but in Asian cultures a bow
is preferred. In South Africa, Turkey, or Arabic countries, a firm handshake
is considered rude; better is a soft, long one. Take the subject of arranged
marriages and you'll find that they are customary in Africa, South Asia,
and the Middle East, whereas a love marriage is more culturally accepted
in America, Canada, and European countries. Another example, cosleeping
(sharing a bed with your children) is practiced the world over, except for
America, Australia, Canada, and Europe. You get the idea. Norms are part
of the way we begin to measure what's acceptable and what's not in society.

The second aspect that helps define normal is the science of *developmental milestones*. Commonly defined as the physical, cognitive, and so-
cial-emotional expectations for children from birth through adolescence,
milestones are divided into four periods:

1. Infancy (birth to three years old)
2. Preschool years (four to six years old)
3. Middle childhood years (six to thirteen years old)
4. Adolescence (thirteen to twenty years old)

Within each period are a series of expected skills and behaviors that
determine a child's growth. Accomplishing such tasks determines if development is on track or delayed. Children achieve these milestones such
as smiling for the first time, rolling over, saying "Mama," bouncing a ball,
learning colors, separating fact from fiction, and developing social peer
bonds through a combination of genetics and psychosocial experiences.

In each developmental period, children move through more evolved and complex milestones, each one building on the ones previously achieved. Knowing these milestones is important not only to help children achieve their optimal developmental potential but also to identify children at risk. It's critical to note that meeting the developmental milestone is more valuable than the age it is achieved. For instance, some children may talk later than others. Some children master social independence before others. The key is the attainment of the milestone.

There are dozens upon dozens of developmental milestones for each period of a child's life—too many to list here in this chapter. Table 1.1 illustrates a small example of some of the skills and behaviors each developmental period involves.

Third in the process of characterizing normal is your child's *temperament*. Defined as an inborn behavioral reaction style, temperament is largely biologically based, is present from birth, and remains stable across one's life cycle.[5] The usefulness of understanding the kind of temperament your child possesses will help you realize the kinds of structure needed to meet life's demands. Your child's temperament will also affect your parenting style, which, in turn, will further shape your child's behavior.[6] Based on classic research on this topic, table 1.2 summarizes nine kinds of temperament dimensions.

Getting an overall picture of how your child moves through each of these dimensions will lead to one of three temperament types as illustrated by the researchers Thomas, Chess, and Birch:[7]

1. Easy—The child with an easy temperament is generally adaptable, approachable, and mild mannered. There is predictability to her rhythms and moods, and she adapts easily to new situations. Expression of frustration is mild or medium in intensity, and she can be readily soothed. Caregivers report that easy-temperament babies are a delight to raise. About 40 percent of children fall into this group.

2. Difficult—The child with a difficult temperament is typically more challenging to soothe, frustrates easily, fusses often, and is feisty. He

Table 1.1. Ages and Milestones

Age Range	Physical	Cognitive	Social-Emotional
Infancy	Strong sucking, grasping, reaching reflexes. Comfortable with routine stimuli; distressed by new stimuli.	Infant begins to "learn" with eyes, ears, hands, mouth, and nose. Has recognition memory for people, places, and objects. Coos and babbles, laughs. Can pay attention and label objects.	Infant forms attachment to primary caregivers, which is the foundation for future socio-emotional and moral development. Shows almost all basic emotions. Develops trust and reliance.
Preschool Years	More complex motor skills; slow, steady growth; toilet training successful.	Explosion of vocabulary, creative and magical thinking. Mastery of learning numbers, colors, letters. Difficulty understanding time values. Solid memory skills developing.	Cooperative but imaginary play. Enjoys peers, takes turns, but may have momentary meltdowns. Wants to please adults. Development of moral conscience.
Middle Age	Use physical activities to develop gross and fine motor skills. Puberty begins for some children at this stage.	More effective coping skills developing. Understands how behavior affects others. Thinking takes on less concrete and more abstract forms.	Begins exploring social roles. Learns adaptation with regard to different contextual situations. Takes on more responsibilities at school/home. Less fantasy play, more team sports, board games.
Adolescence	Growth spurt during this period. Secondary sex characteristics developing. Acclimation to changes in body.	Very busy being introspective. Thinking reaches higher levels of logical, hypothetical, and sequential forms.	Need for social acceptance. Progressive moving away from parents, seeking independence. Sexual exploration. Moods may ebb and flow.

Table 1.2. Temperament Dimensions

Dimension	Description
Activity Level	Level, tempo, and frequency of motor behavior
Biological Rhythmicity	Regularity of biological functions like sleep, eating, and elimination
Approach/Withdrawal	Initial response to new stimuli like people, food, and toys
Adaptability	Ease with which child responds to new or changed situations
Intensity of Reaction	Energy level of response to experiences, mild to strong
Quality of Mood	Balance of behavior pleasant/friendly to unpleasant/crying
Persistence/Attention Span	Continuation of activity in spite of obstacles and time pursued
Distractibility	Degree that external stimuli alter direction of ongoing behavior
Threshold of Responsiveness	Intensity level of stimulation necessary to evoke a response

Source: Thomas, Chess, and Birch (1968)

may be hard to get to sleep for the night; eating and day-to-day activities often have a spirited rhythm. Mood can be disagreeable, with irritability, tantrums, or outbursts occurring. Caregivers report that raising children with a difficult temperament is trying. Understanding, patience, and consistency are needed to help the child, so that a positive adjustment to life's demands can be learned. About 10 percent of children fall into this group.

3. Slow to Warm Up—This child is generally shy, hesitant, or slow to warm up with others. Initial encounters often cause discomfort, but the child slowly adapts. Unlike the difficult child, whose mood is easy to register, there's a slower reactivity, making subtleties harder to recognize as patterns. This child tends to do better if not pressured by others, finding more success when she makes decisions and adjustments at her own pace. Caregivers report that slow-to-warm-up children are not demanding to raise, but they require gentle encouragement. About 15 percent of children fall into this group.

It's been shown that identifying temperament early in a child's life can help stave off behavioral problems,[8] anxiety,[9] and depression,[10] and also help with self-regulation skills.[11] Detecting the type of temperamental style can also clue parents in to the kinds of discipline and structure needed to help

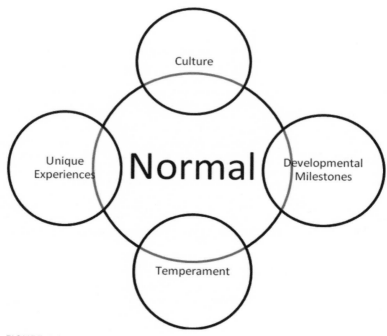

FIGURE 1.1
Elements of Normal

their child adapt to the world. More so than anything else, temperament has a strong association to health, life events, and overall *well-being.*[12]

The fourth and final aspect that is a yardstick for normal are the unique experiences that frame and contour your child's world. These singular moments will influence how he thinks, feels, and behaves—and ultimately shape who he is as a person. What makes this final area so vital is that no two people have the same life story. Your child's personal narrative is incomparably meaningful, so it needs to be celebrated, understood, and valued in its own light. As shown in figure 1.1, the mutual influence and interaction of all these realms—cultural norms, developmental milestones, temperament, and experience—help define normal.

SO, WHAT IS ABNORMAL?

When it comes to detecting mental disorders, there is a general consensus in most of the world regarding what is deemed typical or customary for children as well as for adults. Let's start by defining *abnormal*, which literally means "away from the norm." An abnormal heart rhythm, for example, will vary on an EKG from the anticipated electrical impulses seen in a healthy heart. A summerlike temperature in the middle of winter is considered abnormal because the weather pattern strays from seasonal expectations. With depression, extreme negative moods are not considered a normal experience for children and adults.

Mental health, an important component of well-being, is a level of functioning at which a child can move through the daily demands of life, deal effectively with adversity, work productively, and benefit from social connections. Well-being is a concept that is consistently defined the same way across the world.[13] Behaviors that stray from this state of well-being and cause impaired functioning are considered mental disorders—illnesses characterized by alterations in mood, thinking, and conduct.

Mental illness, like any health issue, will have a range of intensity, activation, and persistence. Disorders can be mild, moderate, severe, or profound; can have an early onset (childhood) or a late onset (adulthood); can be episodic or recurrent; and can fluctuate from situation to situation.

Now that the normal has been defined, let's take a look at a case of mine that highlights why understanding temperament, cultural norms, and developmental milestones are so vital.

CASE STUDY: DYLAN

Dylan, aged three years and two months, was referred by his preschool for evaluation. Concerns were raised regarding his preferences for solitary play over more socialized interactions, poor expressive language, difficulty transitioning from one activity to another, and excessive crying. Prior to Dylan's appointment with me, a full physical examination with his pediatrician revealed him to be in good health, meeting all developmental milestones. A full speech and language evaluation placed him within normal limits for receptive language skills, but just below average for expressive language.

Dylan was a very quiet boy who was small in build. He had brown hair, freckled fair skin, and deep-set blue eyes that disappeared in the folds of his face when he smiled. At the first session, he couldn't immediately separate from his mother, who was sitting in the waiting room, and he clung to her tightly as I tried to encourage him to join me. He finally agreed, although we had to leave the door to the waiting room open a tiny bit to make him comfortable.

Dylan averted making eye contact, and when he did, it was quick and then gone. His movements, though, were gentle and delicate—not the kind of rough-and-tumble of most boys his age. During play-time, he chose Legos, paints, and played at the rice table, making "whooshing" sounds in whispers as he scooped up rice and funneled it into a toy dump truck. When I approached, Dylan didn't refuse my company, but he didn't interact with me or join me in pretend play. When I made loud "vrooming" sounds, crashed my cars, used dialogue in my play, or painted in big, large strokes, Dylan bristled. His reactions seemed to say that what I was doing near him was *too much*. Yet despite the fact that he spoke in one-word answers to my questions—"No," "Yeah," "Uh-huh"—he appeared to enjoy his play. I spent the rest of the session mirroring his play, and this parallel style of interaction allowed him to feel more comfortable. His gaze connected with mine more often, and that's when the smiles began. When a Lego tower he was building swayed, trying to hold its impossible height against gravity, he let out a little laugh. And when it fell to the ground, he clapped his hands in delight, turned to me, and yelled, "Oh, no!"

That was our first real moment of connection. Dylan responded well to my limits and structure of the session. He cleaned up the toys without protest, and he smiled quietly as we tried several times to snap one of the covers to the paints back on. When it finally did, I rolled my eyes, which made him giggle. As the session ended, I asked him to invite his mother into the consultation room, and I watched as he trotted out, grabbed her arm, and said, "C'mon, Mommy." I instructed Dylan to tell his mother what we did, and he sat on her lap and spoke in short sentences, with little physical movement. His mother held his gaze and appeared invested in his every word. The interaction between Dylan and his mother was sweet and tender, and it was obvious that she was attuned to Dylan's need for quiet.

I saw Dylan two more times after that, and each session deepened our connection. He would talk more when asked questions, but he didn't spontaneously initiate dialogue on his own. His play style, however, broadened, with more lively physical movement and animated verbalizations. My evaluation with Dylan's parents revealed a concern over his shyness and preference for alone time; otherwise, they reported he was an easy baby and toddler, sleeping and eating well—"a smart, happy boy—a joy to be around." School consultation showed a different picture, with Dylan's teachers worried that he was a depressed and anxious child. "It's like pulling teeth to get him to do anything," his teacher said. Dylan cried often at school, barely spoke when teachers would ask why he was upset, often refused to eat during snack time, and didn't like participating in group activities.

Formal testing showed that Dylan was a boy with above-average intelligence. No difficulties were found with his moods, thoughts, or other functional areas of his life, except for a moderate impairment in behavior toward others and school/daycare. Dylan was clearly struggling, but not from depression or anxiety. He was an introverted child whose needs were being met at home, but he was being misunderstood at school. He was not depressed.

Recommendations from my evaluation included making sure Dylan's parents and teachers understood introversion—and how it differed from shyness, depression, or anxiety. Introverts require a certain amount of quietness in their life. Introverted children expend a lot of energy being with others, which can leave them feeling tired and setting them into meltdown mode, which can certainly look like depression. So it would be important for there to be a quiet zone for him—and other introverted children in school. For Dylan, when there's too much noise, too many demands, and too many choices, it causes distress. Parenting and teaching that presents Dylan with one task at a time, giving him two choices between things and an area to be quiet and to refuel, will make a big difference for his well-being.

Understanding Dylan's specific needs helped remove the sense of frustration his teacher experienced, and it also helped Dylan feel more secure in who he was, what he wanted, and what he needed in his day-to-day experiences. Understanding child development also helped Dylan's parents embrace his introverted ways instead of being overly sensitive to them.

Children are unique. In order to reach them, teach them, and love them, adults need to recognize aspects of their biology, the textures of their personal experiences, and their special needs. This is why it's crucial for parents to understand child development. When adults become familiar with expected behaviors, personality styles, and predictable experiences, it helps foster a greater awareness of what is normal and what warrants concern.

2

Defining Depression in Childhood

Feelings are defined as emotional experiences, and *mood* is the texture of those experiences.[1] Moods impact our behavior, as well as how we think and feel. To be human is to experience an array of different emotions, from upbeat and hopeful to cool and unconcerned, even frustrated and fearful, in a given day . . . maybe even in a given moment. The heart of human experience beats with moments of joy and flashes of sorrow, and with textures of less potent emotions sprinkled in between.

When our moods ease back and forth along this continuum, we experience a healthy sense of well-being. Most people have good days and bad days, and go on about their life without becoming sidelined. However, there are individuals whose moods crescendo to an overexcited state, plummet toward a hopeless abyss, or cycle between these extremes. People who have these chronic fluctuations in mood don't know a healthy sense of well-being. Their emotional experiences negatively impact how they feel and behave and interfere with their connections to school and work, friends and family. Their general physical health suffers, too. These mood fluctuations stem from an illness called a *mood disorder.*[2]

It has been long believed that although children could experience sadness, they weren't capable of having a true mood disorder. For centuries, depression was an illness exclusively seen in adults. Childhood was considered a time of carefree innocence, when down or blue moods in children were considered "a phase" or "something they would outgrow." Much of the reason for this assumption was the practice of scientists taking adult symptoms of depression and applying them to children. Once research started recognizing that children were not miniature adults and were observed to experience a set of symptoms, science discovered that children can, indeed, have mood disorders.[3]

HISTORY OF CHILD DEPRESSION

Childhood depression, sometimes called *pediatric depression*, has weathered a long journey for recognition. Only in the last twenty years has it been accepted by science as a real disorder. Prior to that, only a small group of individuals believed depression existed in children. The majority of others were of the opinion that children were too cognitively and physically immature to experience depression.

Ancient Greeks first noted depression as an illness in 450 BC. Called *melancholia*, it was seen in adults who displayed a cold and dry disposition—a diagnosis reflected from the theory of an imbalance of black bile in the body. The father of Western medicine, Hippocrates, wrote that melancholia involved an "aversion to food, despondency, sleeplessness, irritability, restlessness and fear."[4] Although later in the first century the Greek physician Aretaeus of Cappadocia described melancholy as having a relationship between the mind and body, little changed in the view of melancholia for thousands of years.[5]

Things started changing in the nineteenth and twentieth centuries when science began branching off from early Greek theories. Studies took a more serious look at how life experiences affected the symptom of melancholy in adults. Epic research in Robert Burton's *Anatomy of Melancholy*, Henry Maudsley's *Physiology and Pathology of Mind*, and Sigmund Freud's essay "On Mourning and Melancholia" furthered the understanding of sadness and melancholy in adults, but they also laid the groundwork for considering depression in children.[6] The fields of neurology, psychology, psychiatry, and pediatrics started tracking symptoms of longing, sadness, and anxiety in children, which helped launch the official discipline of child psychiatry in 1920. Many pioneers such as Melanie Klein, John Bowlby, Anna Freud, D. W. Winnicott, Rene Spitz, and Erick Erickson broadened the field of child depression, detailing theories on trauma, despair, and melancholic reactions in children. But it would take almost a century more for science to truly root itself in the belief that children could, without a doubt, have depression.

The twenty-first century showed a rapid growth of clinical interest in mood disorders in children, influenced by advances in medical technology and the field of neurobiology joining forces with psychology and psychiatry. Evidence-based research studies started streaming in, each one validating aspects of pediatric depression, its symptoms, etiology, and methods of treatment. Scientists agreed that although children had immature and underdeveloped affective (emotional) and cognitive (thinking) skills, depression was something they can experience. Children have mood changes, are capable of having negative thoughts, and tend to show depressive symptoms in more behavioral ways. Examples are joyless facial responses, listless body posture, unresponsive eye gaze, slowed physical reactions, and irritable or fussy mannerisms, just to name a few. Not only did studies confirm pediatric depression but distinctive symptoms were also seen in differing stages of childhood. These results widened the scope of understanding depression in children, and they helped highlight that patterns of depression vary with a child's age.[7]

So the annals of child depression began with a steadfast "no way it could ever be," which shifted to a more thoughtful "oh, yes it can," and then to a postmodern "and it's intricately unique."[8] And now that you have been schooled in its history, let's take a look at the different types of child depression.

UNDERSTANDING CHILD DEPRESSION

You have learned by now that depression in children is not a passing phase. It is a real illness that is clinically recognized and widely treated. One of the best ways to understand child depression is to consider how this illness touches three distinct areas of your child's life: 1) mood, 2) physical health, and 3) self-worth.

Changes in Mood

There are a number of mood presentations that occur in children who experience depression. Whereas sadness and despair make up an adult's depressive experience, irritability and crankiness appear to take center stage in the child. It's important to know that your depressed child may not display this edginess, and instead may appear bored, withdrawn, sad, and unmotivated. Keep in mind that these shifts in mood will likely be accompanied by a lack of interest in things. This is called *anhedonia*, and children show this deflated disposition in play, with sports, among friends, in school, and in other previously loved hobbies or activities.

Changes in Physical Symptoms

Depression will likely impact your child in a physical way, with an increase or decrease in appetite, weight, sleep, and energy. Fatigue can make everyday activities feel daunting for a child, so getting out of bed, brushing teeth, changing clothes, or taking a shower, for example, may take forever to do. What may look like stubbornness in this regard is really the low energy that comes with depression. Another example is frequently seen in adolescence, when teens stop grooming and tend to wear the same clothes over and over again. Though it could be interpreted as rebellious behavior, it likely has its origins in depression. Of great significance for children who are depressed are aches and pains, what are known as *somatic complaints*. Evidence-based studies report depression lowers the immune system and increases inflammation in the body, which raises the susceptibility for sickness, illness, and physical discomfort.[9] Children are often not feeling good physically as well as emotionally.

Changes in Self-Attitude

Depression greatly affects self-attitude and confidence. One of the most alarming aspects of depression is how it distorts thinking. Where positive thoughts once lived there are now negative and self-reproaching beliefs. For adults who have the advantage of having mature cognition, the corrosive effect of depression is extremely difficult to navigate. For the child who has yet to develop problem-solving skills, the dulled thinking that comes with depression is overwhelming, to say the least. Depression will impair a child's judgment, making her feel worthless or unlovable, useless or stupid. She may be overly forgetful, pessimistic, and filled with self-blame. Self-esteem plummets, usually in quiet agony.[10] It's not uncommon for depressed children to make poor choices, feel hopeless, take risks, and deliberate suicide.

SPECIFIC AGE RANGES

We've come a long way from the days in which it wasn't believed children could be depressed. Research now shows that depression can occur at any age, and that symptoms will vary between and among children. Furthermore, rates of pediatric depression *increase* with age, meaning that more children experience depression as they get older. Gender studies tell us that depression equally affects boys and girls in early childhood—though in adolescence, that statistic changes, with girls experiencing depression at twice the rate of boys.[11] Let's take a look at what depression will look like in specific age ranges for children.

- *Babies and Depression (zero to twenty-four months):* I know it's hard to believe, but research has shown that babies as young as six months of age can display symptoms of depression. Much of the research on depression in babies points to biology and biography—the influence of nature (genetics) and nurture (caregiving).

  Etiology for depression in babies is complex, but some examples include structural issues in the *neuroendocrine* and *neurochemical* systems of the brain, which balance stress response and reactivity.[12] Another is the *vulnerability model* that suggests babies with shy, withdrawn, inhibited, or easily upset temperaments are at risk for depression.[13] Then there are *stressful life events* that can impact the attention and care a baby receives.[14] Studies show that the risk of a baby developing depression is about three times higher if he has a parent who is depressed or experiences detached or neglectful caregiving.[15]

According to Dr. Jess Shatkin of New York University's Child Study Center, one in forty babies suffer from depression.[16] Even though babies can't verbally tell us how they're feeling or what they're thinking, there are specific behavioral and physical presentations such as disinterest, lack of responsiveness, poor eye gaze, lethargy, inconsolable crying, sleeping and feeding difficulties, sad facial expressions, and bonding problems. Depression in babies ultimately affects language skills and physical and cognitive development as well. One of the most interesting discoveries in research is that infants identified as depressed continued displaying symptoms of depression even when they were interacting with a nondepressed person—suggesting an already deeply rooted depressive style.[17] I have seen this in my diagnostic work with babies and mothers with postpartum depression. Of all the work I've done in the field of depression, nothing has moved me more than actually *feeling* the depression of an infant as I held them for an assessment.

- *Preschool Depression (two to five years old):* When it comes to studying depression in toddlers and preschool-aged children, no one has done more work than Dr. Joan Luby and her research team.[18] For over a decade, they have been documenting clinical markers for depression in young children, particularly children ages three years old and up. Evidence suggests that approximately 4 percent of preschool-aged children meet the criteria for depression.[19] Studies show that the clinical picture of depression in preschool children has some similar overlaps with typical adult symptoms such as sadness, irritability, and lack of joy. Examples include gloomy or cheerless facial expressions, a cranky or whiny attitude in the presence of others, and not having fun in playtime or with toys.

Other researchers have added to Luby's body of work, noting that preschool depression can sometimes go unnoticed by parents and teachers because symptoms aren't overly disruptive or detectable. It's not unusual for preschoolers to display moody, sullen, or varied behavioral styles—think of the "terrible twos" or the "horrible threes." Another reason this oversight may happen is because some preschool children display "masked symptoms" of depression, expressing guilt, shame, grouchiness, accident proneness, boredom, or aches and pains instead of appearing dejected or sad.[20]

Having worked for many years with this age population, it's quite easy to see how depressive symptoms can be missed. The ages of toddlerhood to preschool are fraught with highs and lows in emotional, behavioral, and learning development. Mastery of skills comes in starts and stops, with chaos and command as children learn to regulate their little bodies, minds, and emotions. Gaps in development aren't unusual, so seeing a child struggling from time to time may not sound any alarms.

What makes seeing depression in preschool-aged children a little more tricky is that this is the age when depression is often accompanied with other co-occurring illnesses or disorders, such as anxiety, ADHD, learning problems, and oppositional and defiance behaviors, just to name a few. This is called *comorbidity*.[21]

- *School-Aged Children and Depression (six to twelve years old):* About 5 percent of children ages six through twelve years old can have depression. What appears differently for children in this age category is a more prolonged pattern of unhappiness, a decline in socialization, sleep problems, and irritability.[22] Also at this age are the beginnings of self-destructive and suicidal thinking, which can come in the form of wanting to run away, frequent physical injuries or accidents, and preoccupation with death. Frequent absences from school as a result of tummy aches, headaches, and other somatic issues are often reported, as are difficulties concentrating, avoiding challenges, resisting new experiences, and a slowness completing tasks at home and at school. Depression can greatly interfere with the process of learning and will be reflected in school performance. If depression is mild, a child may be seen as a slow learner or viewed as possessing underaverage intelligence.

  Social isolation may be dismissed as shyness, disinterest in activities written off as inflexibility, and hypersensitivity misinterpreted as immaturity. Moderate and severe depression at this age tends to be more noticeable, with teachers and/or parents realizing a child is not functioning at an optimal level.

This is a time of rapidly growing language and cognitive skills, as well as the emergence of moral development, when rules, ethics, and the rigidity of right or wrong take center stage. By now, children have enough intellectual capacity and social understanding to realize they are depressed, but they tend to blame themselves for their unhappiness, academic failure, or social disappointments.[23] Studies suggest that boys more than girls express their depression through physical means, such as hitting or bullying, whereas girls convey more vague physical complaints.[24] But don't let statistics be your one and only road map. I've worked with many depressed school-aged boys who were highly symptomatic with physical complaints, and depressed school-aged girls who have kicked some serious ass on the playground.

I have vivid memories of my depression as a school-aged child, struggling terribly from second grade on. My school district used a tracking system to teach, and I was always in the slowest group. I felt lost a great deal of the time and was often made to feel stupid by teachers who had a cruel streak. Teachers who were loving and gentle made it easier for me to be in school, although my academic, physical, and social struggles continued. I was always tired and slow moving, cried easily, and didn't have many friends. I was hypersensitive to everything—the noise in the lunchroom, the bus jostling as it rumbled to and from school. Recess was a sensory overload for me, and I often lingered alone outside or found my way to the library to help stack books or run errands. Once home, I preferred sleeping on the velvet, orange blanket of my bed than going out to play with neighbors. I was a good, quiet kid, but not too smart. That's what my parents thought. That's what my teachers believed. And I don't fault anyone for not recognizing the depressive illness that was slowly swallowing me alive.

- *Adolescents and Depression (thirteen years to eighteen years old):* Recent surveys report that depressive disorders have affected approximately 11.2 percent of thirteen- to eighteen-year-olds; yet only one in five teens get help.[25] As previously mentioned, depression in female teens outnumbers males, with one study reporting a triplefold rate for girls.[26] One of the most somber statistics is that roughly five thousand adolescents who experience depression die by suicide each year.

Teens who struggle with depression display more sleep and appetite disturbances, faulty thinking and impaired concentration, and suicidal ideation and suicide attempts than younger children. Depressed adolescents sometimes seem to be angry rather than sad or discouraged. They are hypersensitive to criticism, and they can come across as annoying or snarky to parents, teachers, and friends. They may show their depression through risk-taking behavior such as cutting classes, stealing, using drugs or alcohol, sexual promiscuity, running away from home, and driving recklessly, just to name a few.

Some adolescents present with a pronounced intensity of despair, dread, and staggering sadness, just like adults. Their depression is readily seen, felt, and registered by others. Other teens are overly irritable, or touchy, but in certain moments, they bounce back and seemingly look and feel okay. This pattern, called *atypical depression*, is the most common form of depression in adolescence—and it can be a challenge to truly diagnose.

Using my clinical skills, I can see that I had atypical depression as a teenager. I had moments of staggering sadness, was irritable, and had learning difficulties—but also smiled, felt good at times, and had moments of academic success. I engaged in rather risky activities, out of character for me—such as skipping school, forging teacher signatures to excuse friends from classes, drinking, drugging, and self-harming in the form of cutting. Fortunately, the recklessness was short-lived as panic and anxiety mixed into my mental health. The co-occurring anxiety disorder may have been a blessing in disguise as the panic that gripped me helped curb my boundary-breaking behaviors. I was afraid of what I was doing, sensing that it was bad and dangerous. I was able to reel them in, and I held the combustible mix from exploding by using a lot of denial ("No, I'm fine, really"), avoidance (sleeping a lot), and distraction (writing poetry and music). For a while, those tools worked to keep my depression from overwhelming me. But in a few years, I would lose the fight.

Table 2.1. Symptom Differences

Signs of Depression in Adults	Signs of Depression in Children
Depressed mood	Irritable, fussy, or cranky
Anhedonia (decreased interest/enjoyment in once-favorite activities)	Boredom, lack of interest in play, giving up favorite activities
Negative thinking, helplessness	Blames self for failures, misperceives peer interactions, socially isolates, resists new experiences
Significant weight loss or weight gain	Failure to thrive, fussy eating, overeating and weight gain (especially in adolescence)
Insomnia/hypersomnia (excessive sleeping)	Difficulty falling asleep, staying asleep, difficulty emerging from sleep, hard to awaken, frequent napping
Psychomotor agitation, restlessness or slowness	Difficulty sitting still, pacing, very slow movements, clingy, little or no spontaneity, overly aggressive or sensitive
Fatigue or loss of energy	Persistently tired, appears lazy, sluggish, reports aches and pains, frequent absences from school
Low self-esteem, feelings of guilt	Whiny, cries easily, self-critical, feels stupid, unloved, or misunderstood
Inability to concentrate, indecisive	Sulks, appears foggy, distractible, poor school performance, forgetful, unmotivated
Recurrent suicidal thoughts or behavior	Worries about death, talks about running away, writing or drawing about death, giving away favorite toys or belongings

It's important that depression in adolescence *not* be confused with the expected angst often experienced by teenagers. Depression goes beyond this, with patterns and symptoms having longer-lasting intervals. Remember, it's not just the presentation of depressive symptoms but also their duration that sets the stage for diagnosis.

WHAT CAUSES CHILDHOOD DEPRESSION?

Research has shown no singular causal root to explain depression in children or adults—or for any mental health disorder. In fact, no illness can truly be described in simplistic terms of *this-leads-to-that*. Instead, multiple determining factors are responsible for why one child is more vulnerable to develop a mental illness than another.

As in my other book, *Living with Depression*, I like to describe the origins of depression as coming from both *biological* and *biographical* influences.[27] This is called the *diathesis-stress model*, and it states that children have, in varying degrees, genetic and biological predispositions for developing mental illness. Another way to explain this is to say the mind and the body are not separate entities, but they are interconnected and influence each other.[28]

We as adults, and children too, have built-in propensities. These hardwired vulnerabilities are called *diatheses*—and they include genetics, our neurochemical makeup, and the structures of our psyche. The other part of this model looks at the overwhelming feature of life events and environmental experiences, otherwise known as *stress*. This biology-biography model suggests that having a propensity toward developing depression alone is not enough to trigger the illness. Instead, a child's diatheses (vulnerabilities) must interact with stressful life events in order to prompt the onset of the illness. Not every child who has a propensity for depression will develop it. This is nature and nurture in a most unique interaction.

I've written before that taking a look at my life history shows the diathesis-stress model in action. As a baby and young child, my temperament was passive and quiet. I wasn't demanding and didn't protest when I was uncomfortable—or when things were stressful. Family discord and a series of losses and separations left me frightened, alone, and emotionally adrift. I didn't fight to free myself from toxic situations and accepted the fate of my circumstances. This is called *learned helplessness*, a hallmark indicator of depression. As I grew older, my symptoms worsened. Distorted thinking and poor judgment led to learning problems, academic failure, risk taking, and sexual abuse. I closed down, isolated myself, and descended into a pattern of negative and hopeless thinking. I was emotionally battered and physically spent. Back then I didn't know that all of the traumatic experiences I weathered alongside the genetics of my depression set up the perfect storm for mental illness. And when it arrived, it hit me at gale-force speed at age nineteen: major depressive disorder with suicidal intent.

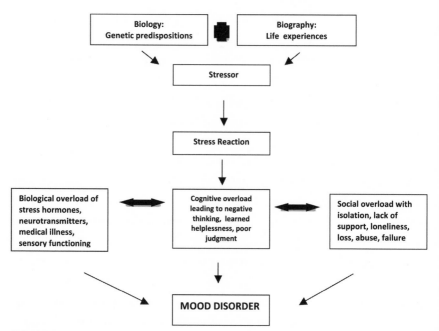

FIGURE 2.1
Diathesis-Stress Model

TEN QUESTIONS TO ASK YOURSELF

Now that you know more about child depression, it's time to ask yourself a few questions. Doing so helps identify if your child is struggling with a mood disorder, and it will also raise your awareness of what this experience means to you.

1. *Is my child free from any medical illnesses at this time?* This is always my first go-to question. Ruling out that your child isn't experiencing any medical or physical illness is vital in diagnosing depression. Make sure your child has a recent physical with relevant lab work to rule out illnesses such as diabetes, anemia, and hypothyroidism. Illnesses such as these can mimic depression, as their symptoms include fatigue, listlessness, irritability, and sleeping and eating problems.

2. *Is my child's behavior age-specific?* Remember, different age ranges involve expected levels of irritability, moodiness, and inactivity. If you're not sure what developmental behaviors are anticipated for your child's age, a quick search on the Internet will help.

3. *Has my child gone through any recent traumatic event(s)?* Next up, take a moment and review you and your child's life to see if any significant changes have occurred. Things such as a loss, death, divorce, a school change, hospitalization, car accident, or a new babysitter, for example, can overwhelm a child with a propensity for depression. These events or experiences are called *triggers,* and they often set into motion a traumatic reaction.

4. *Does my child's behavior interfere with age-related tasks?* If your child is irritable or sad, is it interfering with the learning of new tasks? For example, babies will be slow to develop motor and language skills, school-age children will struggle with school or social connections. Teens may flunk classes or resist planning for what happens after graduation. Review how your child is meeting these expected goals.

5. *What is the intensity of these behaviors?* Once you've noted the suspected symptoms of depression, see if you can sense their force or magnitude. Is your infant's crying weak or strong? How long is she crying? A few minutes? Hours? Does your toddler quickly move from sullen to happy? Is your teenager deeply angry or just mildly irritable? What does that look like? When we yardstick these symptoms, we bring a more accurate picture of depression to the diagnostic table.

6. *How long have I noticed them?* This may be easy for some parents to recognize, while others may have a harder time. Don't worry if you can't recall an exact time length for your child's symptoms. What's important is estimating whether your child's thoughts and/or behaviors are new ones (days or weeks) or longer in their presentation (months or years). The length of time will lead to specific diagnoses, so that's why you need to ask yourself this question.

7. *What is the duration of these experiences, and do they happen in other places?* Now that you've noted the intensity and length of your child's symptoms, it's time to analyze where they happen. Do they only occur only at home? Do they occur in school? Is your baby the same with you as he is with others who spend time with him? What about with friends? On the school bus? With extended family? The diagnosis of depression looks at the range of where symptoms occur. This is called *pervasiveness.*

8. *Does my child's symptoms remind me of anyone in my family?* Genetics create the blueprint for who we are, but they are not a guarantee of who we become. That being said, studies show that more than 25 percent of children who have a parent with depression will be diagnosed with the disorder.[29] So take a look at yourself and your partner. If either of you has a diagnosed mood disorder, this is important to note. Be gentle and curious as you ask these questions. Widen the scope and look at relatives. Does your family lineage have depression, anxiety, or any mental illness? This is not about assigning blame. This is about recognizing how heredity can influence depression.

9. *At this moment, am I worried about my child?* Most parents are quite worried about their child by the time they're sitting with me in my consultation office. In fact, I'd say that nine out of ten parents have a good sense of what's going on with their baby, child, or teen. Rare is the occasion that a diagnosis surprises parents. At least, that's been my experience working with families. So it's okay to be worried about your child. It means that you detect something. It means you're attuned to your child. And it means that you are a vital piece of the diagnostic procedure. So trust your instincts and share your concerns.

10. *How will I feel if my child is diagnosed with depression?* Putting a name to a set of experiences can be an empowering moment. It can validate what you, as a parent, have been seeing in your child. You can feel a sense of relief in knowing there's a name for your child's experiences— and that there's a plan of action in place. But getting a diagnosis can also leave you upset and unsure. Be aware that a diagnosis causes a variety of unexpected thoughts and emotions. Reactions such as shock, disbelief, fear, anxiety, guilt, sadness, grief, and anger are part of the experience of receiving a diagnosis of depression—or a diagnosis of any illness for that matter. Give yourself time to process what this means to you. Explore and express with trusted loved ones or a professional. Your acceptance of your child's depression will play a vital role in her treatment and *recovery.*

CASE STUDY: LENA

"She's eight years old. What's she got to be depressed about?" Lena's father asked.

Lena's mother wrinkled her brow. "I don't understand. You're telling us she *really* needs to keep up the therapy?"

Lena was referred to me from the social worker at her new elementary school. Lena's teacher noticed from the beginning of the school year that Lena often wore some of the same unclean clothes over and over again. In the halls, she walked with rounded shoulders, didn't have many friends, and seemed to be a "very unhappy girl." When her hygiene began to decline, the teacher contacted Lena's parents, but not much changed after that contact, so the teacher asked the social worker to look into things. Lena shared with the social worker that she didn't really like school, but it was better than staying at home. Concerned, the social worker evaluated for neglect and/or abuse, but she found no evidence to call in Child Protective Services.

Lena, a girl of average height and weight, spoke with a slight accent, and she frequently averted eye contact. She told me she was the first to be born here in the United States, and that much of her family moved here from Europe when they were adults. Lena was an only child and was supervised by her grandfather because her parents "worked a lot."

It was clear from the start that Lena and her family were financially challenged but that there was a great deal of love in the home. However, with her parents working most of the time, Lena felt alone and unsupported, especially when it came to "girl" things. She told me learning in school was easy, but she didn't really think anyone in her class liked her. She wasn't bullied; it was more like she was ignored. She didn't have cool clothes. She didn't have fun things like a phone or an iPod, and she didn't talk like everyone else. Despite not fitting in, Lena reported that she liked being in school better because at home she got bored a lot.

Over the course of sessions, I learned that although Lena had a close, loving family, there were gaps in parenting and cultural styles that created feelings of insecurity and low self-esteem. There was little empathy and compassion, and Lena's parents often treated her as if she were much older—demanding more independence and less "whininess" from their young child. The move to a suburban neighborhood from the urban setting she was used to added to her loneliness. Lena was already used to talking herself out of hope—phrases such as *why bother*, *it doesn't matter*, and *I don't really care* were already part of her repertoire.

It was hard to schedule appointments with Lena's parents because they worked long hours and weekends trying to make ends meet, so a lot of communication occurred on the phone. Although her grandfather cooked and cared for the entire family, he didn't venture beyond the confines of the home and local supermarkets—which made Lena's world a very small one. Getting Lena to my office for an appointment was like asking him to trek to the far ends of the earth . . . but her grandfather got her to me for every session.

Treatment for Lena was all about helping her adjust to her new school and neighborhood. I offered the "girl" guidance she was so desperately looking for—and slowly she came out of her shell. She especially enjoyed thumbing through the catalogs of clothes that regularly came to my house, and she seemed very moved that I tucked them aside for her. She loved coloring and playing dress up—and she would sometimes go the entire session with a tiara on her head. Lena's teacher reported an improvement in her overall presence at school. She was groomed and clean and raised her hand in class to contribute more often. The social worker noticed one day that Lena had a new outfit on, and that she walked tall in the hallway. "Like seeing a flower bloom," the social worker said to me.

Treatment for Lena's depression was going well, but it was often thrown a monkey wrench by her parents. They had a hard time believing Lena needed therapy. She had a roof over her head, food on the table, and was loved. What more could she need? To heal Lena's depression, her parents had to understand that their daughter needed much, much more. It would be difficult, if not impossible, to shift Lena's negative self-talk without her parents' support. As is often the case, parents who don't believe in therapy convey to their child that the changes being made aren't acceptable.

Try as I might to help Lena's parents understand the issues at hand, they felt blamed, judged, and were reluctant to work with me. They viewed therapy as a stigma, and they didn't like the idea of Lena sharing stories about her family. Putting a name to their daughter's struggles didn't give them comfort. In fact, it was just the opposite. It seemed to make them angrier and less compassionate about Lena's struggles.

After several months of treatment, Lena began missing appointments. It was not because she didn't want to come but that her grandfather "couldn't get her there." I spoke to Lena about how it sometimes takes time for adults to face their own worries and fears about things—and that we should be prepared that our work might be interrupted as time went on. It was hugely important to counter the effects of her parents' reluctance to deal with her needs, wants, and desires. Lena already had a fragile view of herself and was prone to hopeless thinking. So we worked hard on helping Lena see that her family's minimizing of the work we were doing was a result of their own insecurities—and not that she was unworthy.

As predicted, Lena's parents stopped treatment. But Lena and I arranged for her to talk with the social worker at school to keep working on changing her dysfunctional thinking styles. I like to think that Lena continued moving forward, but because I was no longer in the picture, it's hard to know for sure.

The case study illustrates how pediatric depression requires both an understanding of its origin and a supportive environment from parents to reduce symptoms. Without them, conflict and confusion will likely flood the already turbulent waters a family navigates when a child has depression. The hope for Lena is that psychotherapy, though short in its duration, showed her how sadness, depression, loneliness, and despair *can* and *should* be expressed, and that there's no shame in feeling such emotions; there are ways to lessen how they hurt inside—and that she can find her way with others if she can't find encouragement at home. And perhaps most of all, it helped her to not be angry at her parents for their lack of support, but to try to understand their limitations.

3

Diagnosing Pediatric Depression

One of the questions I'm asked most often is "Why diagnose a child at such a young age for depression?" It's a good question—and an important one. Diagnosis of *any* mental disorder at a young age is subject to debate. No one wants to "pathologize" childhood behaviors such as tantrums and moodiness—or slow-to-reach developmental milestones. It's easy to think of them as "just a stage" of development or as something a child will outgrow. But what if taking a casual approach to these troubling behaviors results in missed opportunities? What if they're not stages?

Studies show that early detection of an illness always benefits treatment.[1] With a thorough evaluation, you'll learn if your child's behaviors are the result of a true clinical disorder, place him at risk for possibly developing a clinical disorder, or are age appropriate and something he'll outgrow.

Now, I understand that the stigma of mental illness is strong in our culture. And I know how a "diagnosis" can turn into a "label"—reducing a child to a set of stereotyped misperceptions. But putting off assessment *now* for evaluation *later* can do more harm than good. Emerging research shows that diagnosing early interrupts the negative courses of some mental illnesses, improves recovery, and increases the likelihood of complete *remission*.[2] As a parent, you'll have time to learn how to deal with stigma and to find ways to make sure your child is seen for "who she is"—not for "what she has." What's important right now is finding out whether or not your child has depression.

Let's start by first understanding the diagnostic procedure. The word itself—*diagnosis*—is derived from both Latin and Greek origins, meaning "to distinguish or discern." The goal of diagnosis in children is to identify *symptoms* as problems, not *children* as problems.[3] So when we talk about pediatric depression, the goal of diagnosis is to achieve the following:[4]

1. To diagnose the presence and extent of behavioral problems
2. To identify a child's specific abilities and skills
3. To identify a child who may be at risk for depression
4. To identify a child who has depression
5. To determine appropriate intervention strategies

The diagnostic assessment requires you, as a parent, to be part of an important team. Along with professionals from the fields of medicine, mental health, and education, you will seek out the what-and-why reasons your child is struggling. Sometimes a diagnosis will be easy to obtain. Other times, it might be hard to determine. Whatever the outcome, you and your team will collaborate to find solutions to help your child.

HOW DIAGNOSIS IS DONE

Advances in molecular biology, genetics, and brain research are leading the development of genetic and blood tests to diagnose mood disorders. In the near future, these tests will be the tools of choice. In the meantime, diagnosing depression in children is a ruling-out process.

Given that many medical illnesses can look like a mood disorder, a multistep approach for diagnosis is recommended. The first link in the diagnostic chain is for your child to have a comprehensive medical examination. A pediatrician needs to assess your child's physical health and rule out any illnesses or diseases that could present as depression. This wide-ranging assessment should include a physical exam, medical history, and blood laboratory studies. Sometimes illnesses such as diabetes, hypothyroidism, anemia, and Epstein-Barr virus—and even side effects of over-the-counter and prescription medicines—can mimic the symptoms of depression. Getting a reliable diagnosis of depression requires you to be open and honest, so in addition to being candid regarding your child's physical health, it's important to share any known family history of mental illness, as well as any drug or alcohol use, with your pediatrician.

Once your child's medical history is deemed noninfluential for causing depression, your next stop will be a consultation with a mental health practitioner. In this setting, a thorough evaluation of your child's presenting behaviors will be the focus. The clinician will be assessing your child's behaviors at home and/or school, as well as the timing, presentation, and duration of depressed symptoms. The relationship between stress and depression is well established, so you will be asked if any significant changes, losses, or traumas have occurred in the recent past—and if chronic personal, family, or financial stressors press on your life.

The mental health practitioner will need to spend time assessing your child. This shouldn't be a breezy ten minutes followed by a formal diagnosis! I always worry when I hear a parent say they walked into a doctor's office and seconds later walked out with a prescription. A systematic diagnosis is very involved, often taking one to three sessions. The clinician will examine your child's mental status (intellectual, emotional, psychological, and social functioning), paying particular attention to irritability and mood. For older children and teens, risk taking, suicidal thinking, and personality traits will be assessed. And just as the clinician asked you about recent traumas and stressors, so, too, will your child be asked.

Some clinicians use a structured clinical interview to diagnose, while others invite standardized depression scales. There are many different kinds of depression scales, too many to mention here in this chapter, but here are a few that are often used:

- Beck Depression Inventory[5]
- Children's Depression Inventory[6]

- Conners Comprehensive Behavior Rating Scales[7]
- Infant/Toddler Symptom Checklist[8]
- Inventory of Complicated Grief[9]
- Millon Adolescent Clinical Inventory[10]
- Pediatric Emotional Distress Scale[11]
- Reynolds Adolescent Depression Scale[12]
- Reynolds Child Depression Scale[13]
- Trauma Symptom Checklist for Young Children[14]

Another link in the diagnostic chain is to evaluate for comorbidity. As previously mentioned, pediatric depression is often accompanied by other coexisting issues, such as anxiety, learning disabilities, and substance abuse, just to name a few. If coexisting disorders are present, treatment recommendations will address each of them.

After gathering all the data from interviews, sessions, and medical history, a clinical diagnosis will be reached using a diagnostic manual. In the United States, the classification system used to diagnose mental illness is the *Diagnostic and Statistical Manual of Mental Disorders* (DSM)[15] and the *Diagnostic Classification of Mental Health and Developmental Disorders of Infancy and Early Childhood: Zero to Three* (DC:0–3).[16] In all other countries, the World Health Organization's *International Classification of Diseases* is used.[17] After a clinical diagnosis is determined, a treatment plan will be offered for your child's depression.

TYPES OF PEDIATRIC DEPRESSION

Let's review how different kinds of depression can "look" for children. One of the best ways to illustrate this is to view mood disorders as having two categories: *unipolar* (in which mood roots itself in a depressive state) and *bipolar* (in which mood fluctuates between the lows of depression and the highs of mania). These mood disorders are illustrated in figure 3.1.

If a child is in the midst of a unipolar experience, the ebb and flow of behaviors, thoughts, and emotions tend to linger in the low ends. The bipolar experience involves the margins of sadness, too, but it differs in that

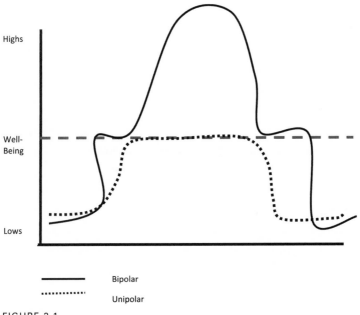

Highs

Well-
Being

Lows

——————— Bipolar

·············· Unipolar

FIGURE 3.1
Mood Disorders

it also elevates to the high ends of mania. Often, a pattern of moods can be observed—a cycling back and forth from sadness to excitement. This is called a *mood swing*.

Now that you have a working understanding of these disorders, let's summarize each one in little more detail.

UNIPOLAR DISORDERS

At any given time, up to 15 percent of children and adolescents have some symptoms of depression.[18] They may differ in intensity and duration, leading to different diagnostic categories. Here are five unipolar disorders that a child may experience.

- *Major depressive disorder (MDD)* is the *most serious* of the unipolar disorders.[19] For children, specific symptoms have to occur for at least two weeks. Children may experience varying degrees of unshakable sadness, loss of interest, slow thinking, poor judgment, and, in some cases, suicidal thinking. Major depressive disorder can be mild, moderate, severe, or profound, and episodes can last for several months—and reoccur if not treated. MDD can be experienced at any time, but a subtype is only experienced during seasonal changes. This kind of MDD is called *seasonal affective disorder (SAD)*, and it affects approximately 3 percent of children.[20] SAD often occurs during the fall and winter months when decreased sunlight and colder weather set in. But it's important to note that SAD can present during the seasonal change of spring and summer, although this is less frequently observed. Suicidal risk is high with any mood disorder, but it is highest with major depressive disorder.

- *Dysthymic disorder (DD)* is a less severe form of depression. With DD, symptoms are more chronic and persistent, with children feeling sad or irritable not for months, but for years. For adults, DD symptoms must be present for two years for diagnosis. For children, the qualifying time is one year.

Dysthymic disorder can be harder to detect because the depressive experience has a slower and more subtle trajectory. Children with DD aren't obvious in their depressive presentation; rather, they present with a glum exterior, with slow-moving ways and bouts of crankiness. Often children with DD live so long with their low-grade depression that they don't really know they're depressed. This was me as a kid. I lived so long with my chronic depression that I just thought that was the way life was supposed to be. It never occurred to me that I could feel happier, cry less, or be less foggy and groggy.

Children who have dysthymic disorder are at risk for having major depressive disorder at the same time.[21] This is called a double depression. Generally, a double depression is triggered by significant life events. I know about double depression professionally because I've worked with many children who've experienced this. But I personally know about double depression because I experienced one as a teen when the pressures of college became too much for me. The one-two punch from my dysthymic disorder crashing into a major depressive disorder knocked me out cold—and sent me spiraling into a despair that resulted in a suicide attempt.

- *Adjustment disorder with depressed mood (ADDM)* is *the most common depressive mood disorder* in children and teenagers.[22] Symptoms start within three months of an identifiable stressor, like a school change, marital conflict, divorce, a fight with a friend, or a new babysitter. This mood disorder is a reactive one, in which a life stressor presses on a child's emotional and social functioning. What is highlighted here is that a child's emotional experience exceeds what would be considered a normal reaction in the face of a trauma. Symptoms of ADDM are *not* caused by bereavement, and they do not last longer than six months after the stressor has stopped.

- *Adjustment disorder related to bereavement (ADRB)* is a disorder that a child develops six months after a significant death, when unrelenting grief and sadness hasn't improved with time.[23] Normally, grief doesn't need formal clinical intervention. Time and support from loved ones help heal the stages of grief. However, there are children whose grief becomes chronic and debilitating over time. For these children, there is a challenge in making sense of the *permanence* of the loss.[24]

- *Depressive disorder not otherwise specified (D-NOS)* is diagnosed when depressive symptoms do not meet the criteria for MDD, DD, or an adjustment disorder. D-NOS is generally offered when the reasons for presenting depressive symptoms are unclear, but warrant treatment. The most well known in this category is *premenstrual dysphoric disorder (PMDD)*. The symptoms of PMDD are remarkably similar to those of MDD. On average, menstruation begins at age twelve, so girls and teens can experience PMDD, which is defined as severe depressive symptoms that arise before a menstruation cycle.

BIPOLAR DISORDERS

Bipolar disorders are less common than unipolar ones in children. As mentioned before, there are two different sides to the disorder—depression and mania. In 40 percent of children who are diagnosed with a bipolar disorder, their illness presented with a major depressive disorder first.[25] There are three bipolar disorders that comprise the depressive experience for children and teens.[26]

- *Bipolar disorder I (BD-I)* for a child may include periods of depression with fatigue, forgetfulness, helplessness, and hopelessness washing out his world. He may move into a state of high activity, in which excitability, overreaction, and irritability take center stage. Called *mania*, a child may have so much energy that he doesn't want to eat or sleep; talks loudly, pressured, and fast; and behaves in reckless, impulsive, or promiscuous ways. There can be a broadening of his sense of self, perhaps thinking he is able to do more—or be more—than he really is.

  It is very important to know that bipolar disorder in children can look like attention deficit hyperactivity disorder—a neurobiological disorder in which impulsiveness, restlessness, and distractibility cause pronounced difficulties. Because these two disorders share symptoms, misdiagnoses often occur.

- *Bipolar disorder II (BD-II)* is characterized by at least one major depressive episode and an observable hypomanic episode. *Hypomania* is a milder form of elevated mood than is mania and does not necessarily impact daily functioning. Sometimes called "soft bipolar disorder," the symptoms are less intense that bipolar I, but are more chronic.

- *Cyclothymic disorder (CD)* is a mild form of bipolar disorder, in which a child experiences episodes of low-level depression, followed by periods of intense energy, creativity, and/or irritability. These cycles are usually short in duration and less strong in their intensity. Like dysthymic disorder, many children and teens don't realize they have a serious issue going on. For CD to be diagnosed, mood swings need to be experienced for two years for adults, and one year for a child.

  Cyclothymia is one of the least diagnosed bipolar disorders because depressive symptoms aren't usually incapacitating for a child, nor are the erratic high moods. It isn't unusual for cyclothymic disorder to be missed entirely or misdiagnosed as bipolar II or borderline personality disorder (a mental illness in which a pervasive pattern of instability in interpersonal relationships, self-image, and emotions occurs). Left untreated, CD can worsen and turn into bipolar disorder I.[27]

SUBCLINICAL ISSUES

Sometimes the diagnostic evaluation may not yield a diagnosis. This means your child's thoughts and behaviors didn't meet the criteria for a formal clinical disorder. On occasion, the diagnostic threshold isn't reached, though symptoms of depression do, indeed, exist. When this happens, the term *subclinical* is used to describe test findings.

What research tells us about subclinical symptoms is that they are risk factors for developing a full-on disorder.[28] But fret not, because there is gold in this diagnostic nugget. Simply said, discovering these symptoms early can help derail the oncoming disorder that may be barreling down the pike for your child. Emerging research shows that preventive interventions such as shoring up your child's strengths, working on shifting negative thinking patterns, and re-educating learned helplessness styles to more proactive ones interrupt the formation of clinical disorders.[29]

THINGS TO REMEMBER

A proper diagnosis of *any* mental illness hinges as much on the diagnostician as it does with presenting symptoms. That being said, it's crucial to find an experienced mental health professional that understands pediatric depression. Also keep in mind that putting a diagnosis to a set of experiences can be empowering. It validates a reality that was long held suspect. When I was first diagnosed with a major depression disorder as a teenager, I felt relieved and released. Everything I had experienced and suffered through finally made sense. However, as a practitioner I know that delivering the diagnosis of pediatric depression can swing parents to the other extreme. It's important to recognize that the process of diagnosis, any diagnosis, can elicit strong reactions. Some elements to consider:

- *Uncertainty:* When an evaluation ends with a diagnosis, it also signals the beginning of an emotional journey. That can leave a parent feeling afraid, alone, and anxious. The unknown can be scary, so ask yourself if you're feeling worse because you're unsure about what comes next.
- *Grief:* A diagnosis can be experienced as a loss, too, leaving you feeling traumatized. Research shows that receiving a diagnosis moves a person through the five stages of grief: denial, anger, bargaining, sadness, and acceptance.
- *Stigma:* Explore your internal reactions to your child's diagnosis. Are you feeling shame about having a child who is struggling with depression? Do you think you failed in some way? Do you worry how loved ones will respond if you share your diagnosis?
- *Comparison:* Some parents move through acceptance of a mood disorder diagnosis more readily than others, so don't compare yours to anyone else's. Just remember that with the diagnosis of depression comes the hope for recovery.
- *Process:* Remember to give yourself time to adjust to your child's diagnosis. Little by little, address your concerns so you can ease your worries. Be it alone, with your spouse, or with the support of others, realize there is more to your child than her depression.
- *Disclosure:* Moving through all of this on your own or with your spouse can be a tall order. Consider sharing your thoughts and feelings with a trusted friend or perhaps a therapist.

In this chapter, you've learned how pediatric depression is diagnosed and the different subtypes of mood disorders. The following case study shows how certain illnesses can make detecting depression a slippery slope.

CASE STUDY: KEVIN

Kevin, a fifteen-year-old high school student, had been in treatment on and off since the second grade. First diagnosed with attention deficit hyperactivity disorder at age six, he was prescribed Strattera to offset his impulsivity, distractibility, and hyperactivity, and he was in biofeedback therapy for behavioral changes. Throughout elementary school, he struggled in class subjects and was prone to temper tantrums. Psychoeducation testing was recommended, and Kevin received special education services such as extended time limits, a quiet place to take tests, and extra support in the classroom. In middle school, he became depressed and oppositional—outwardly refusing to go to school—and was placed on home tutoring. Frustrated at how things were going, Kevin's parents sought a new therapist and psychiatrist, believing that his current treatments weren't really helping. With cognitive behavioral therapy and a new medication regime, Kevin began to feel better and returned to school.

In high school, Kevin discovered academic strengths in writing, and he enjoyed the more independent ways students were encouraged to behave. He also excelled in sports, finding a particular love of long-distance running on the track team. He seemed to have outgrown his "temper tantrums," but he still described himself as moody—an adjective his parents wholeheartedly agreed with.

Kevin found his way to me after a week of sleepless days and nights resulted in a physical crash of fatigue. He refused to get out of bed, and he missed a couple of days of school. In what Kevin described as *just being pumped writing a term paper*, his parents as well as his physician saw something else. Kevin's dad, Greg, said, "It was as if he was like the Eveready Battery Rabbit, going and going and going." Kevin's mother, Sheryl, noticed how fast he talked and how enthusiastic he was about everything. Kevin's physician thought he was in the midst of a manic episode, and considered bipolar disorder as the cause. After working with Kevin for a few sessions, I concurred with the physician's thoughts. Assessment indicated symptoms that met the criteria for bipolar disorder I. A change in medication helped stabilize Kevin's moods, and he really found his stride in talk therapy, becoming more aware of his behaviors and thoughts.

At first, Kevin's parents were angry that the other professionals missed diagnosing him accurately. I understood their frustration, because no parent wants to think their child had to suffer unnecessarily with wrong treatments or medications. I tried to help them see that diagnosis can *only be certain* of what is behaviorally presented—and back when Kevin was a young boy, testing pointed to ADHD. I educated Kevin's parents on how childhood bipolar disorder is tricky to identify, especially in young children, and that if I was working with them back then, I might have found ADHD as well. Of course, it's little consolation to say such things, but I wanted Greg and Sheryl to not allow blame and shame to stop their momentum in helping Kevin.

Sometimes a wrong diagnosis happens. It leads to needless expense, misdirected effort, and worries of side effects from unnecessary medication. It is traumatic when this occurs. Time has to be spent undoing the original diagnosis and learning to understand the new diagnosis. The emotional impact of misdiagnosis tends to hit parents harder than it hits children. For Kevin, he took the medication change and the treatment adjustments as if they were a simple turn on a street. He liked that the misdiagnosis explained why he kept having trouble all those years. In a way, it left him feeling stronger and more confident in his abilities.

Kevin has been doing very well, and he wants to come off his mood-stabilizing medication. This is a common thought for anyone, especially kids, when they feel good. My work with Kevin right now is to help him understand that his bipolar disorder requires him to manage it daily. After recently going to the movies with his girlfriend to see *Silver Linings Playbook* (a movie that highlights bipolar disorder and what it takes to live with it), he tells me he "gets it." But I know that it will be a journey for him that has its ups and downs—literally as well as figuratively.

4

Treatments for Pediatric Depression

Once diagnosis is completed and recommendations made, you are likely to consider traditional treatments for your child's depression. Traditional treatments are so termed because they are the go-to techniques that have evidence-based research to back them up. Generally speaking, traditional treatments fall into two major categories: psychological and medical.

PSYCHOLOGICAL TREATMENTS

Psychotherapy is the treatment of emotional conflicts through the use of talking and communicating with a trained professional. Also known as *talk therapy*, psychotherapy is practiced by psychologists, psychiatrists, social workers, mental health counselors, and psychiatric nurse practitioners.

There are many different types of talk therapy, each one working from a unique model of mind and behavior. Though these treatments may differ in approach and technique, they all share the same goal: to reduce your child's depressive symptoms. Let's take a look at several kinds of different talk therapies, presented here in alphabetical order.

- *Attachment-based family therapy (ABFT)* treats pediatric depression by using a family system approach. This means that you and your child, as well as other family members, will be part of the treatment.

Essentially, ABFT focuses on looking at how aspects of the family environment can worsen or help depression. For you, parenting skills and the quality of your parent-child dynamic will be addressed. For your child, ABFT will help teach alliance building, *affect regulation*, and ways to enhance self-concept.[1] ABFT can be used with toddlers, preschoolers, older children, and teens.

- *Behavior therapy (BT)* is a psychotherapy that focuses solely on your child's actions or behaviors. Typically, your child will meet with a therapist once a week to look at what kinds of behaviors reinforce the depressive symptoms. Is she focusing on the negative aspects at school instead of the positive ones? Is she stuck in a loop of negative social reinforcement from friends? Do you as a parent respond with great concern when things are bad, and gloss over the happier moments? Behavior therapy helps sharpen your child's observational skills. She will learn the power of consequences, and how well-being can come from changing behaviors. Behavior therapy is recommended with school-aged children and up—it is not usually used with younger children because of their limited verbal abilities.

- *Behavioral activation (BA)* is an offshoot of behavior therapy, and it looks at avoidance as being the leading cause of depression. BA works to make your child aware of the inactivity and patterns of avoidance in his life so that he can modify his behavior. When you avoid, you become disconnected, leading to loneliness and self-doubt. Skill building involves "activation strategies"—techniques that will get your child connected and involved with others.[2] You and the therapist will monitor your child's progress with charts and rating scales in this short-term therapy.

- *Cognitive-behavioral therapy (CBT)* works a bit differently than behavioral treatments, believing that *thoughts* as well as actions worsen depression. CBT emphasizes how your child's inner dialogue (core beliefs) and the repertoire of her behaviors keep depression from healing.[3] Does sadness leave her thinking she's not good at anything? Is the fatigue she feels making her believe she's lazy? Does she think the world is not a safe place? In this therapy, your child will meet once a week with a therapist to begin identifying the dysfunctional belief systems she uses on a daily basis. The goal here is to correct unrealistic beliefs and behaviors by replacing them with more realistic attitudes. Essentially, changing how she behaves and thinks will change how she feels.

- *Dialectical behavior therapy—for adolescents (DBT-A)* includes aspects of changing behavior and adds the Zen Buddhist principles of acceptance and mindfulness to the mix. DBT-A is a short-term, sixteen-week program through which your teen will learn how to set behavioral targets, work through dialectical dilemmas, and find a healthy middle ground.[4] Often, your participation in this treatment is required, with family sessions built in in addition to the individual sessions your teen will have with the therapist.

- *Interpersonal therapy (IPT)* is another short-term psychotherapy, usually consisting of a forty-five-minute weekly individual session for about three months. Children and teens can undergo this treatment, which involves a warm but straightforward look at their interpersonal lives. Like detectives, your child and the therapist will identify negative social habits and emotional blind spots—and develop new skills to offset depression.

- *Mindfulness-based cognitive therapy for children (MBCT-C)* is a group treatment therapy for school-aged children aged nine to thirteen years old. This twelve-week program teaches children how to manage depression with breath meditations and how to use their senses to measure internal and external experiences, self-care, and kindness, among other things.[5] Parents are encouraged to be co-participants and be involved in their child's home instruction exercises.

- *Parent-child interaction therapy* is a form of play therapy that actively revolves around you and your child. There are three aspects to this treatment. The first looks at how you effectively praise and positively reward your child, the way the two of you play, and other parent-child dynamics. The second component teaches you how to discipline and set limits with your child. The third teaches you how to help your child regulate his or her emotions, particularly sad and depressive ones. Research shows this treatment is highly effective for toddlers, preschoolers, and young children.[6]

- *Play therapy* is an excellent treatment for very young children who experience depression.[7] As little ones find it hard to express their thoughts and feelings in words, play becomes the mode for communication. Be it toys, clay, paint, sand tables, or action figures, your child will learn through play how to problem solve, modify behaviors, regulate her moods, learn new ways to relate to others, and develop stronger self-esteem.[8] Sessions are generally forty-five minutes, once a week, and they are individually based. Sometimes parents are invited in to play sessions, so wear comfortable clothes.

- *Psychodynamic short-term psychotherapy (PSTP)* is an insight-oriented therapy for children and adolescents that focuses on self-awareness, motivation, and meaning in your child's life.[9] The immediate goals of PSTP are to label feelings and learn new behaviors by creating *corrective emotional experiences*. In this treatment, a therapist meets with your child once a week to reduce depressive symptoms only but also to understand the underlying issues that might be contributing to it.

MEDICAL TREATMENTS

Relatively speaking, parents seem to share a universal response to the idea of medical treatment for mental illness. It usually begins with a breathy sigh, followed by a jaw-dropping, wide-eyed shrug of the shoulders.

The thought of introducing these kinds of interventions to a child is scary and unnerving—and I totally understand the fear that comes with that. Talk therapy is an *external influence* that modifies thoughts and behaviors, whereas medical treatments are *internal influences* that modify thoughts and behaviors. It can make for some hesitant decisions.

One way to help understand the recommendation for medical treatment for your child's depression is to remember that a mood disorder has *neurobiology* as its origin. Though research shows talk therapy can change levels of dopamine and serotonin, sometimes more intensive medical treatments are necessary to help shift this neurobiology.

Research shows that your beliefs regarding medical interventions will have a direct effect on your child.[10] If you are uncertain and afraid, it may trickle down to him. If you feel hopeful and confident, he will receive that message. Before embarking on any of these interventions, it's a good idea to read, research, talk with others who have been through this, and make sure you and your partner are on the same page.

I have worked with hundreds of families, many who started out fearful in the beginning of this journey. With time, they learned that their decision to add medical interventions was not only helpful but also life saving.

- *Pharmacotherapy:* Thousands of years ago, plants, flowers, and minerals were sourced for their medicinal purposes. They soothed cuts and bruises and healed sick children. It may be hard to believe, but the practice of pharmacotherapy is THE oldest of the traditional therapies for mental illness. What modern science has done is to borrow from ancient pharmacotherapy to create bioactive compounds to treat mental illness. Sometimes referred to as *drug therapy*, pharmacotherapy changes the neurochemistry in your child's brain and body to heal depression. Pharmacotherapy is not just a long and hard-to-pronounce word—its mere mention frightens many parents. But if carefully researched and professionally guided, using medicine can be a viable way to address your child's depression.

  In this treatment, you and your child will work with a trained medical professional who specializes in the management of mood disorders. The pharmacotherapy process involves a thorough medical history, one that will take up your entire first consult. While you're there, the specialist will match your child's symptoms with relevant medications and begin him on a small dose.

  At first, you and your child will have scheduled appointments within weeks of starting the medication. As time progresses, the dosage may remain the same or increase based on your and your child's reports. If side effects are intolerable, a change in medication may be necessary. However, once depressive symptoms are reduced, you won't need to be seen as often.

Keep in mind that pharmacotherapy *and* psychotherapy are often used together in a treatment plan. So you will have one professional monitoring your child's medicine and another professional teaching her skills via talk therapy.

- *Inpatient hospitalization* is recommended when psychotherapy and pharmacotherapy aren't successfully reducing your child's depression. Another reason for inpatient hospitalization may be because your child is in a very fragile state, contemplating suicide, or in the throes of an agitated mania. The safe setting of a hospital is vital for stabilizing your child.

Sometimes inpatient hospitalization can be planned; that is, you, your child, and the professionals involved decide to take this route because current treatment is not yielding good results. Generally, I call ahead and get the admission process started to ease the transition. In an emergency situation when your child is suicidal or self-destructive, there often isn't time to set up admission. In this event, getting to the nearest hospital's emergency room is the primary goal.

Many inpatient hospital wards are more like college dormitories than the sterile, white secure units portrayed in movies. Single or double rooms with beds and desks are the norm. There's a community room with welcoming chairs and sofas, a television, and recreational activities—and phones for keeping in contact with loved ones. It's true that most of these hospital zones are locked and there are rules that need to be followed—such as visitation times, permissible clothing, and accessories, just to name a few. These precautions keep your child and others safe and enable the staff to manage the floor with continuity.

The main purpose of seeking inpatient treatment is to intensify all aspects of therapy. Medication is monitored more closely. Talk therapy occurs on a daily basis, either individually, in group, or with family members. Once your child is feeling better and stabilized, she'll be discharged. Long stays in hospital settings are rare. When she leaves, she may have the ability to continue care in a *partial hospital program*. In this kind of treatment, she will go on with her daily routine at home and/ or at school, and in the late afternoon she will return for daily supplemental therapies.

TREATMENT-RESISTANT DEPRESSION

Sometimes a child or adolescent can experience a depression so problematic that more intensive medical treatments have to be considered. This type of depression is called *treatment-resistant depression (TRD)*. Research defines TRD when your child's depression does not ease after trying two or more trials of antidepressants.[11]

It can be an overwhelming experience to realize that interventions aren't helping. Everyone feels frustrated—you, your child, and the professionals in your team. The time invested in talk therapy and medication may make you feel it was all a gigantic waste of time. But clinicians never feel that any of the work was for naught. In fact, it is just the opposite. It indicates that your child needs more than traditional science and what its interventions comprehend. Cutting-edge scientific research brims with data on depression, but Big Pharma and medical technology haven't been able to keep up with these discoveries. And that's what you and your child need to understand to help make this easier to move through.

The most vital piece in treatment-resistant depression is not to let too much time go by trying a varied assortment of antidepressants—or allowing months morph into years taking on different kinds of talk therapies. The cycle of trying and failing over and over and over can make children feel deeply despondent about their illness. Moreover, it can make you feel frightened for your child's future. But working with a TRD specialist can ease your worries and help your child find hope again. Let's take a look at these often misunderstood, but life-changing, treatments.

- *Electroconvulsive therapy (ECT)* is only considered in depressed adolescents after the failure of three or four medication trials and at least one trial of psychotherapy hasn't helped.[12] Refined from its early beginnings, ECT is no longer the fearsome treatment pictured in television and films. In fact, ECT is performed while your child is comfortably asleep under short-acting anesthesia. A team of anesthesiologists, nurses, and medical doctors perform the procedure in a medical suite.

    Essentially, ECT is the process by which electrical currents are passed through the brain to create a brief seizure. This shifts signal pathways and neurotransmitters in the brain that eases depression. ECT treatments are generally given every other day for up to twelve treatments—and take about fifteen minutes to perform. There can be side effects, which include headache, nausea, and muscle soreness and short-term memory loss.

- *Repetitive transcranial magnetic stimulation (rTMS)* is a treatment for adolescents in which a coil-like tool is positioned around your child's head to apply short, magnetic pulses to target specific areas in the brain. rTMS is much less invasive than ECT, but it seeks to have the same results—shifting neurochemistry and signal pathways of the brain. rTMS has minimal side effects, such as headache, tingling, and light-headedness, but they are reported to reduce quickly.[13]

    Unlike ECT, rTMS is performed while your child is awake, often in a doctor's office. The treatment takes about forty minutes, and daily treatments are recommended for about a month. There is no down time, so your child can resume her activities right away.

- *Vagus nerve stimulation (VNS)* was initially used for the treatment of epilepsy in both children and adults, but VNS has shown to improve depression in adolescents eighteen years and older.[14] VNS involves the surgical implantation of a device under the skin by the collarbone that sends electrical pulses through the vagus nerve—a pathway that regulates mood. This procedure is done in a hospital under anesthesia. Adolescents who have undergone this treatment report almost immediate reduction in depressive symptoms with no side effects in memory or thinking. Typical complaints are soreness, irritation, and infection at the surgical site, as well as nausea. Battery power lasts three to five years and will require replacement, which means undergoing surgery again.

THINGS TO REMEMBER

If your child doesn't respond to traditional and/or medical treatments, you may feel worried that relief is elusive. Keep in mind that the treatments of today were once the experimental practices of yesterday. So there will always be hope. In fact, a stream of experimental treatments for depression have been making news. Recent studies show great promise using the anesthetic drug *ketamine* for treatment-resistant depression,[15] as well as *transcranial direct current stimulation (tDCS)*, which is similar to ECT, although it is done while awake.[16] And then there is *deep brain stimulation*, similar to vagus nerve stimulation, although it is more target specific,[17] and *personalized medicine*, in which a person's unique genetic makeup is used to create specialized medicine, making the treatment of depression work more successfully and with little or no side effects.[18]

When making the decision for treatment for your child, be sure to find professionals who specialize in mood disorders. Always, ALWAYS, get a second opinion once a treatment plan has been designed. I cannot encourage this enough. As a parent, you want to feel as confident as possible so that, in turn, your child will feel assured of the path taken. Become familiar with the interventions—their risks and benefits, pros and cons, short-term versus long-term side effects, and cost and accessibility—so you can make an informed decision.

Before we leave this chapter, take a look at the following case study. Within this story is an all-too-common experience many children have when treatments don't offer relief. It is presented here to show the importance of how a support team of expert clinicians and caring family members can help find hope.

CASE STUDY: THERESA

Theresa often stopped in for counseling with the school psychologist in middle school, but she was referred for outside psychotherapy when her depressive symptoms became more intense. She was a young teenager when I met her for consultation. We instantly clicked. Theresa was smart and thoughtful, a beautiful girl with expressive brown eyes and a sweet smile. She loved music and animals. And she loved her family. But somewhere near the surface was a melancholy—and I sensed its dark contours.

Her medical reports were negative for any illnesses, but her family history was significant for depression. In fact, Theresa's mother openly discussed her chronic and intense struggles with depression, which included use of tricyclic antidepressants.

My assessment with Theresa yielded an Axis I diagnosis of dysthymic disorder. A treatment plan was designed using cognitive behavioral interventions to shift negative thinking as well as insight-oriented techniques to build greater self-awareness. From the start, Theresa worked hard in sessions and was invested in learning ways to diminish her depression. But as treatment progressed, Theresa encountered many challenging life stressors, including the death of a friend. Talk therapy was unable to bring the intensity of her depression to a more manageable level, so medication was introduced. Working along with Theresa's family, her school, and the psychiatrist wasn't enough to keep a major depressive episode from occurring, however. This double depression proved dangerous, as she became self-destructive and suicidal, requiring inpatient hospitalization.

Once admitted, a change in medication and daily therapy helped to stabilize her mood. Theresa bounced back, returned to high school, and resumed her work with me. But gains made were short-lived. A pattern emerged—one that Theresa, her parents, and I recognized. We discovered that the second change in medication wasn't yielding significant symptom relief—much like we saw in the first go-around with antidepressant medicine.

Prescribing antidepressant medication in dosages that are too low and for lengths of time that are too short are common causes of treatment failure. Theresa's psychiatrists and I considered this possibility with her first experience with medication. This time around, Theresa's prescribing doctor took a more intensive tact, shifting the timing of her medicine and slowly increasing the dosages to find a therapeutic level. The process demanded a lot of time and tolerance. A tall order for anyone, let alone a teenager. But Theresa accepted this challenge. And we all held our breaths to see if the increased dosage of this new medicine would do the trick. It didn't. And soon her dysthymia worsened again, setting off another major depressive episode with suicidal intent.

Theresa's second hospitalization was longer and more intensive. She attended a partial hospital program after discharge and began working with another psychiatrist. Theresa's medication was changed once again—and added to the mix was a second medication to boost the effect of the antidepressant. This is called *augmentation therapy*, and although it offered Theresa more relief than *monotherapy* (one antidepressant), it didn't bring her depressive symptoms to a level at which she could function adequately.

Given that Theresa's mental health struggles were so similar to my own, I couldn't help but feel crushed when treatment failed her again. I wanted her to feel relief. I wanted her to find hope. Together with her family and the new psychiatrist, we talked about treatment-resistant depression and contemplated using electroconvulsive therapy (ECT). Theresa and her family researched long and hard before agreeing to go forward with ECT. It was really quite amazing to watch as her mom and her dad worked to understand the grip depression had on Theresa, how they collaboratively asked questions, weighed options, and considered what-ifs.

After the first few ECT treatments, it was clear that their decision was the right one. Theresa reported feeling better. For the first time in years, her bright eyes and sweet smile gleamed again. Now, this is not to say that she didn't have difficult moments or trying times. She did. And one of the ECT side effects of short-term memory loss frustrates her to this day. But what changed the most was the intensity of her depression. No longer was she a prisoner, chained to a never-ending sentence of quiet agony and despair.

Theresa's work with me ended not too long after her ECT treatments finished and her life journey took her out of state. Now in her thirties, she keeps me up to date with the goings-on in her world through email and Facebook—and an occasional visit to the office when she's in town. She continues psychotherapy as a way to deal with the chronicity of her depression and has found a successful medication regime. Like me, she will have to take medication for the rest of her life. And Theresa's okay with that. She has found a way to live as well as she can in spite of having depression—and she reminds herself of where she is now and how different it is from where she once was.

I always tell Theresa that she was the most courageous kid I ever worked with—which she brushes off with a roll of those expressive brown eyes of hers.

5

Holistic Approaches to Depression

Depression is an experience of depletion. As I child, I distinctly remember feeling worn down, hollowed out, devoid of enthusiasm or vitality. I didn't realize, back then, that the biological aspects of depression were dulling my senses, draining me to a level where I took in very little around me. I lived in a featureless existence—one that I understand far better today as both a clinician and a patient in recovery. But as a young girl, I thought the world was just a muted place that had little to offer—and I had little to give back in return.

Research shows that our moods are affected the most by what we take in through our senses.[1] What we see, smell, taste, touch, and hear activate every cell of our being, setting into motion a series of neural cause and effects.[2] And it's not a linear, one-domino-touches-another-and-then-another kind of experience. Our sensory system, a collective tour de force of cell receptors, firing neurons, and surging chemistry, gives way for emotions and thoughts to be born. And this complex symphony creates the human experience.

When depression occurs, the sensory system deteriorates.[3] For example, senses become dull. Neural pathways slow down. Important feel-good neurochemicals wither in production. What depression does to children, as well as to adults, is flatten the human experience. But feeding the senses

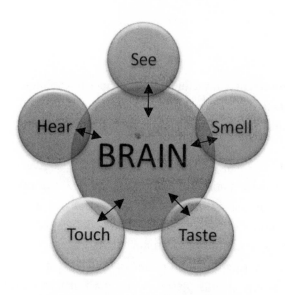

FIGURE 5.1
The Brain and the Five Senses

in the right ways can help balance neurochemistry, revive sluggish neural pathways, and bring greater well-being to your child. And research agrees, showing that refueling your five senses with complementary and alternative medicine (health approaches not considered traditional or conventional) offers psychological, social, and behavioral benefits.[4]

SIGHT

The very first thing a depressed child needs to have is light. The data on sun and natural light holding powerful holistic benefits for depression is vast. It has been my professional opinion, as well as my personal experience, that in order to lift the veil of depression, one has to be able to see the light—literally and figuratively. So open the curtains. Draw the blinds. Let the sun's light spill into your child's room. Encourage your child to move into a pool of sunlight. If she has enough energy, see if getting outdoors is possible, even if it's for just a few minutes.

Light is responsible for turning on the brain and the body. Light enters through our eyes, moves through the retina, and signals the *hypothalamus*, which regulates mood, sleep, and appetite. Light also activates the *pineal gland*, a tiny, pea-shaped brain structure that essentially runs our body clock, producing the hormone *melatonin*. When we live in darkness, the pineal gland produces too much melatonin, making us sleepy, fatigued, and listless. One of the greatest benefits of being in sunlight is that it helps to even out melatonin production—and keep our body clock running smoothly.

If abundant sunlight is not available, you can create it for your child with artificial light. *Bright light therapy* has been shown to suppress the brain's secretion of melatonin almost as well as natural sunlight. Bright light therapy uses a spectrum of blue light in the morning hours. If bright light therapy is done late in the afternoon, your child's body clock will become disrupted—and so will her sleep cycle. Your child needs to get at least twenty minutes of bright light for its positive effects to take place. Keep in mind that the bright light need not be directly in front of her, but within the room, so her retinas can register the luminescence. Once your child can move from a listless state of depression, start to reteach her *to truly see, not just look at things.* Help her learn to drink in the colors and textures of the world. Linger in nature's uplifting beauty.[5] Take notice of the budding leaves on trees, the tinted blooms of newborn flowers, or the way the sun's hue deepens its orangey glow as spring arrives. Teach her by modeling your own observations of people, animals, and things in your world—how they look and move, and what makes them unique and beautiful.

And speaking of color, don't forget to bring it into your child's life for greater health and balance. Color is a well-documented mood lifter, and it has been used to help arthritis, bulimia, cancer, wound healing, and, yes, depression. If your schedule is too chaotic to manage big ways to bring color, such as painting a room or installing a color-lighted showerhead, ask for help. Little ways to invite color can include buying brightly colored towels, vivid clothing, decorative items, toys, stuffed animals, and even colored flowers from your yard or local supermarket.

The practice of using color to heal is called *chromotherapy*, and it has been around for thousands of years.[6] Some of the first to use this ancient healing method were Egyptians, who built large glass rooms, called solariums, where the sun's light would flood an ill person with color. Chromotherapy uses the visible spectrum of colors, calling on their electromagnetic properties to heal illness. Blue is calming, violet simulates imagination, red is invigorating, orange is optimistic, yellow brings lightness and fun, and green summons harmony. Find what colors work for your child and invite them into her room and into your home. Consider encouraging her to bring a crush of color to school as well, not just with clothing but also with colorful supplies or backpacks. Brightly colored pens and pencils, key chains, locker wallpaper, mood lighting, and vibrant magnets can elicit uplifting feelings. Light in the school environment has been trending in research, notably with the Phillips Lighting Company using a bright light therapy approach to classrooms called School-Vision.[7] This surface-mounted lighting structure houses four different light settings: "energy," a blue-hued light that is used in the morning when students are sleepy and still awakening to the day; "normal," which is switched on when pupils are coming in or out of a class; "calm," which has a red hue for breaks or rest times; and "focus," a bright white light that is used during exams and presentations. Research has shown that using this type of light therapy increases the learning, concentration, and test performance of children. Ask your school if this evidenced-based program can be incorporated in your child's school.

Another way that sight can enhance mood is the notion of space. Research shows that high ceilings and open spaces aid in the recovery of depression. Studies have shown that dwelling in rooms with low ceilings and confined environments reduce cognitive performance, memory, and dampen moods.[8] So make sure to expand the space in your child's day. Most people don't have vaulted ceilings and feng shui décor, but with a little elbow grease, you can create the illusion of space by decluttering rooms so the line of vision is elongated and fluid. Make sure to tend to her bedroom and at least another area in the house where she spends a good deal of time. If arranging a clutter-free, open area isn't possible, there is always the outdoors. No matter the season, encourage her to spend some time outside. Making sure to incorporate open, sacred places to heal depression is a great tool.

A further strategy to use the sense of sight to enhance well-being is to look at photos that are sweet, colorful, or playful in content. I'm always on the lookout for pictures that bring forth feelings of warmth, happiness, awe, and inspiration. I call this antidepressant photo therapy. Cute animals. Beach scenes. Maybe it's muscle cars, the latest NASA Hubble telescope photos, or a music heartthrob. Find whatever kinds of photos make your child happy, and set her imagination afire or tickle her funny bone. Another sight-oriented tip is to collect uplifting or motivational sayings. Fortunes from cookies, blurbs from magazines, poster quotes, or even sayings and proverbs from the Internet are all great ways to get active with words of wisdom. I've been known to cut, paste, and print those that I find online and tack them around my home for when I need a motivational boost. I also fold them up and pile them in a basket in my office, adding a surprise element for a child who's grabbing one for inspiration. Consider collecting them with your child, making them screen savers on her computer, or threading them into a slide show to offset declining moods. Make a collage together and paste them on a poster board, or quietly leave them in unconventional spaces around the house for her to find, like the linen closet, her dresser drawer, or her shoe.

When it comes to my sense of sight, I use all these holistic approaches. I get at least fifteen minutes a day of natural sunlight, and I have a portable blue light box for when the sun isn't out. I incorporate color, take advantage of wide open spaces, and take the time to see, not just look at, what's going on in my world.

SMELL

Smell is the most nostalgic of all your senses. A certain aroma, scent, or fragrance can immediately remind you of an experience or a memory. This is because smell takes a direct route to the limbic brain, where emotional memories are processed. Smells can bring forth good feelings or bad ones. So when your child is experiencing depression, or may be heading for a bout of depression, it's important to learn which scents give him an emotional boost.

Using the sense of smell to help offset depression is called *aromather-apy*. Like chromotherapy, aromatherapy is an ancient practice that has volumes of research backing its claims. The science of scent shows that the right kinds of fragrance activate brain structures responsible for mood, focus, and thinking—the *hippocampus* and the *amygdala*. More specifi-cally, scents such as bergamot, basil, or peppermint have been shown to increase concentration. If you want to lift mood, try lemon, vanilla, or lavender. If your child is struggling with the sadness of a broken heart, citrus or minty scents such as orange, lemon, spearmint, and grapefruit can help minimize the hurt. For calming and relaxing, try scents such as jasmine, chamomile, lemongrass, and rose.[9]

Often, boys are slow to consider using aromatherapy, believing it to be too girly or flowery for their tastes. A little history teaches them that a male French chemist, René-Maurice Gattefossé, began aromatherapy. And later, in World War II, male surgeon Dr. Jean Valnet used essential oils to heal soldiers wounded in battle. There are many mood-boosting scents that are less flowery or citrusy, such as sandalwood, patchouli, cy-press, cedar, ginger, and black pepper.[10] The key is to find a scent that your child likes and encourage its use to help bring about well-being.

You can buy aromatherapy items in the form of essential oils, incense, candles, potpourri, wax melts, sachets, linen sprays, diffusers, vaporizers, and heating beads at your go-to local bed and bath stores or online at spe-cialty shops. Spray a beloved scent on your child's sheets and pillowcase, splash some essential oils in his bath or steamy shower, dab some on his temples, chest, or other pulse points, or make a sachet out of a funky fab-ric of his choice. I don't recommend that children directly use candles or incense, but that doesn't preclude you from overseeing their use. On the cheap, take a pot of water and add cinnamon, vanilla, or peppermint ex-tract. Simmer for a few minutes and then turn the stove off. The scent will travel through the house, offering a welcoming lift to all. Aromatherapy at home is an easy thing to do, but when it comes to school, check in with his teacher to find out if such holistic measures could be too distracting to the other students.

Aromachology is a new trend that gets its name from blending aroma and psychology. Personalized scents are created in oil, candle, or necklace form—and used as an emotional support system to create a personal "scent bubble." Less expensive and more attainable than a designer scent is to allow your child to discover an over-the-counter cologne or body spray that sparks his sense of smell. Long ago, perfume was considered solely an adult experience, but nowadays a wide and varied fragrance market is available for children and teens. In my practice, I recommend parents and kids shop together to ensure that the fragrance choice is developmentally age appropriate.

Another way to help revitalize the sense of smell and improve his mood is to use air filters and ionizers. Studies done on ambient indoor pollutants are linked to irritability, lethargy, physical illness, and decreased cognitive functioning, just to name a few.[11] We spend nearly 90 percent of our lives indoors, so cleansing with a HEPA air cleaner helps not only your child's mental health but also his physical health. Ionizers are small machines that produce a flow of negative ions into the air. Different from positive ions, which are produced by climate-controlled air, televisions, and computers (causing sleepiness, irritability, and weakness), negative ions balance serotonin levels, thus improving mood. Not only have negative ionizers been shown to reduce depression, but they also relieve stress, improve concentration, and boost energy.[12] Such devices can be pricey, so cost may not allow for one to be in every room of your house. If so, consider placing at least one combination air filter/ionizer in your child's bedroom, and another in a part of the house he most often dwells, such as the playroom, den, or kitchen. Other forms of *negative ion therapy* include wearable personal ionizers, negative ion sprays, feng shui waterfalls, and salt lamps, but do keep in mind to note negative ion output levels for best results.

Much like a depressed child needs to have the curtains drawn for light, don't forget to open the window as well. Studies have shown that individuals who experience *green space*—that is, fresh air and nature—have lower rates of depression, anxiety, and poor health than those who don't.[13] Additionally, stilted, unventilated air has a surplus of positive ions, and

as previously mentioned, will create a sleepy and fatiguing effect. Keeping the window open for fresh air on a sunny day is always a welcoming
experience, but after a rain shower is the best of all. Negative ions are at
their highest then.

During my depressive episodes as a child, I had experiences with many
of these scent-altering methods. My father, who was a chiropractor in the
1960s and 1970s, used essential oils in his practice and would often invite
me to use them. I can still remember how the eucalyptus and peppermint
scents instantly awakened me from my dulled and dark moods. My mom
would soak clean washcloths in a pot with either orange peel and vanilla
extract or fennel seeds and honey, wring them out, and rest them on my
forehead when I had crying spells. I played in the rain—and open win-
dows abounded in my childhood home. I still use essential oils, favoring
lavender and sandalwood now, and I use candles, potpourri, incense, and
linen sprays almost daily. I sit outside for bouts of fresh air, and I use
air filters and ionizers in my home and office. I know they help me feel
grounded and balanced, because if I forget them when traveling, I feel a
big difference—and the difference isn't good.

TASTE

Research has shown that your child's sense of taste may diminish when
depressed due to the shift in serotonin and dopamine levels. For some,
this may mean a loss of appetite. For others, it may shift their appetite
into overdrive. If your child is like me, and her appetite never, ever dimin-
ishes, be mindful that certain foods will worsen her mood. Sugary foods
and starchy carbohydrates will give her a quick, feel-good rush, but in the
long run, it will irritate her blood chemistry and digestion. If your child
is barely eating, when hunger finally hits, it's wise to refuel her with good
foods. So let's take a look at the many foods that have been shown to help
in the recovery of depression.

1. *Ancient grains* are called "ancient" because they've been around, un-
   changed in their wholesomeness, for thousands of years. These foods
   are high in protein content, have more calcium than milk, and are rich

in vitamins and minerals. Research reports that ancient grains such as quinoa, millet, teff, amaranth, spelt, barley, and kamut are complex carbohydrates, which take longer to digest, so they don't cause spikes in blood sugar that can create roller-coaster moods. *Nutritional Concerns:* These grains are a whole-grain alternative for children who are allergic to wheat. But for those who cannot tolerate gluten, steer away from barley.

2. *Folate* is a water-soluble form of vitamin B9 that the body requires from food for cell growth. Folate gets its name from the Latin word *folium,* for "leaf." Research has long connected folate in the synthesis of serotonin. Studies show that many depressed children and adults often have low levels of red-cell folate and serum folate. Folate can be found in leafy green vegetables and certain dried beans such as black-eyed peas, brown rice, and lentils, as well as fruits such as oranges and bananas. *Nutritional Concerns:* Foods high in folate can cause gastro-intestinal stress. Too much folic acid supplements can result in a rash, so make sure a pediatrician oversees your child's usage.

3. *High flavonoid foods* have plant pigments that color flowers, fruits, and leaves. Flavonoids are so prized because their pigments offer anti-inflammatory and antioxidant benefits. Research shows that flavonoid-rich foods are associated with better performance in cognitive abilities and in strengthening the immune system. Flavonoids also help improve mood and decrease irritability and fatigue.[14] So don't be afraid to plate up with foods such as apples, blueberries, dark chocolate, deep red grapes, tea infusions, and tomatoes. *Nutritional Concerns:* These can become harmful if taken in supplemental form and should be monitored by your child's physician.

4. *L-theanine* is an essential amino acid derived from tea leaves that works to balance the production of dopamine and serotonin. Furthermore, research on L-theanine has shown that it can induce alpha waves, the brain waves one achieves when meditating. It has been shown to reduce heart rate, increase focus, and lower blood pressure, as well as promote periodontal health and reduce cavities. L-theanine is found primarily in green tea and matcha (finely milled green tea powder).

Table 5.1. Recommended Dietary Allowance for Children, By Age

Food	0–6 mos	7–12 mos	1–3 yrs	4–8 yrs	9–13 yrs	14–18 yrs
Ancient Grains	*	*	1.5–3 oz	2–4 oz	3–5 oz	306 oz
Folate	65 µg	80 µg	150 µg	200 µg	300 µg	400 µg
High Flavonoids	*	*	*	*	*	*
L-Theanine	*	*	*	4–6 oz	4-6 oz	4-6 oz
L-Tryptophan	*	*	91 mg	133 mg	238 mg	340 mg
Magnesium	30 mg	75 mg	80 mg	130 mg	240 mg	360 mg
Omega-3	*	*	0.7 g	0.9 g	1.0 g	1.3 g
Proteins	9.1 grams	13.5 grams	13 grams	19 grams	34 grams	52 grams
Vitamin B-12	0.4 mcg	0.5 mcg	0.9 mcg	1.2 mcg	1.8. mcg	2.4. mcg
Vitamin D	400 iu	600 iu	600 iu	600 iu	600 iu	600 iu

*No RDI has bveen established for this, so please consult with your physician.
Source: Office of Dietary Supplements, National Institutes of Health (2005)

Nutritional Concerns: Green tea has been deemed safe and beneficial for children in limits of four to six ounces a day by the American Dietary Association, but it is not recommended for toddlers and infants.[15] As with anything your child ingests, make sure their intake is being monitored by a pediatrician or registered nutritionist.

5. *L-tryptophan* are amino acids that are used by the brain to help produce serotonin. Once in our body, tryptophan is converted to 5-HTP (5-hydroxytryptophan), which is a compound that synthesizes serotonin.[16] And since our bodies can't produce tryptophan on our own, we need to get it nutritionally. Clinical trial studies have shown that adding tryptophan to a diet can lift mood. Not only has tryptophan been used to help depression, but it has also reduced insomnia, anxiety, headaches, bruxism, and premenstrual dysphoric disorder, just to name a few. You can find amino acid L-tryptophan in animal protein as well as avocados, bananas, Brussels sprouts, cantaloupe, collard greens, figs, oranges, potatoes, and spinach, and in nuts such as almonds, cashews, and pecans. *Nutritional Concerns:* Tryptophan does not come in herbal supplement form; however, supplements of 5-HTP for children have been used, but with varying results. Therefore, it is recommended that you consult with your child's pediatrician to monitor dose and effects if you choose this approach over getting tryptophan from food choices.

6. *Magnesium* is involved in hundreds of biochemical reactions in the body. Some of them include regulating blood pressure, heart rate,

sugar levels, metabolism, and keeping our immune system in tip-top shape. What's significant is that research reports magnesium is often low or deficient in children and adults who experience depression. More specifically, magnesium plays an important role in the production and synthesis of serotonin, so low levels will affect well-being.[17] Magnesium can be found in foods such as legumes, vegetables, whole grains, nuts, soy, and seafood, as well as cereals, milk, and chocolate. *Nutritional Concerns:* If your child has kidney issues, do not incorporate magnesium without working alongside your physician. For those without kidney issues, side effects of magnesium can include slight gastrointestinal distress. Whether incorporating magnesium with over-the-counter supplements or directly through food, be mindful of the recommended daily requirements for your child's age.

7. *Omega-3 fatty acids* are called essential fats because they can't be manufactured within the human body and therefore must be consumed through diet. Like protein makes up our muscles and calcium our bones, essential fats make up about 60 percent of our brain. But not any fat will do. We need a special fat, called *docosahexaenoic acid* or *DHA*. Surveys have shown that the more fish the population of a country eats the lower their incidence of depression.[18] The reason why? Fish contain high amounts of omega-3 DHA, which has been shown to increase blood flow to the brain, balance dopamine and serotonin levels, and enhance mood, just to name a few. Research has found that increasing DHA consumption also boosts gray matter in the amygdala, the hippocampus, and the cingulated gyrus, three areas of the brain associated with mood. Feeding your child foods such as salmon, nuts, eggs, and olive oil will help invite healthy amounts of DHA and may help reduce depression.[19] *Nutritional Concerns:* Various studies have noted a manic risk if too much omega-3 is used in supplement or nutritional form for teenagers. As with any of these recommended food tips, make sure you consult with your doctor.

8. *Proteins* contain amino acids that aid in the creation of endorphins—a family of neuropeptide neurotransmitters that influence our mood. Proteins such as pork, poultry, lean meats, eggs, and fish take longer

to metabolize, which stabilizes blood sugar and leads to a more satis-
fied feeling after eating. High sugar levels can leave your child feeling
irritable, fatigued, and moody—and hungry a short while later. More
importantly, eating lean proteins replaces *catecholamines*—a neurotransmitter that keeps us feeling upbeat—and balances serotonin.
Nutritional Concerns: Too much protein in a child's diet can cause de-
hydration and intestinal irritation. Balance and moderation are key.

9. *Vitamin B12* is involved in every cell of your child's body. It is significantly important for brain and neural pathway functioning, metabolism, and blood production. Studies show a connection between low
levels of vitamin B12 and symptoms of depression.[20] A blood test can
help determine if your child is lacking in this important nutrient. As far
as food is concerned, vitamin B12 can be found in seafood such as snap-
per, shrimp, and scallops, and in fermented vegetables such as miso and
tofu. Just like omega-3 and folate, vitamin B12 dietary supplements can
be useful. Injections, sublingual tablets, or sprays are also available as
well. *Nutritional Concerns:* Too much B12 from supplements can result
in headaches, stomachaches, dizziness, and diarrhea.

10. *Vitamin D* works along with melatonin to even out your child's
sleep/wake cycle and regulate his immune system. Vitamin D also
lowers the production of *cytokines*, which are proteins that increase
inflammation. A number of studies have shown cytokines to be
a possible risk factor for depression.[21] Low vitamin D levels have
been implicated in depression in children and adolescents,[22] and
in the seasonal affective disorder subtype as well.[23] Vitamin D can
be found in foods such as shiitake mushrooms, eggs, fortified milk,
fortified grains, and oily fishes such as salmon, cod, catfish, tuna,
and mackerel. About 90 percent of vitamin D gets absorbed through
sunlight, so help your child get out in the sun. Blood tests are available to determine if your child has a low or deficient vitamin D
level. *Nutritional Concerns:* Be watchful of overloading vitamin D by
making sure you work with your child's pediatrician and stay within

recommended guidelines for your child. Side effects of too much vitamin D include nausea, constipation, dry mouth, and headache.

Once your child experiences a lift from his depressive symptoms, see if you can help him use his sense of taste to call forth positive feelings. Studies show that even small moments of flavor sensations can lift mood. So show him how to nurse a delicious cup of hot chocolate or swirl a piece of candy slow and long in his mouth. Whatever foods or beverages he enjoys, help him learn how to take delight and savor the experience.

I have always been taste oriented, and I find feeding this sense to be an easy task. When at my worst depressive moments, I found taste to be the only comfort I could call on to soothe me. Hot vegetable soup and sweet fruit got me through many a depressive episode as young adult. I've long practiced what I preached, eating well, taking supplements, and balancing many of these foods into my cooking repertoire. I often borrow from neuropsychologist Fernando Gómez-Pinilla, telling many of the children and families who live with depression that "food is like a pharmaceutical compound that affects the brain. The more balanced you make your meals, the more balanced will be your brain functioning."[24]

TOUCH

There are many positive effects that come from touch, being touched, and moving your body. For example, touch reduces the production of the stress hormone, *cortisol*, eases irritability, soothes loneliness, lowers blood pressure, calms heartbeat, and surges the bonding hormone, *oxytocin*.[25] Touch is a reaction to contact, and it is an especially meaningful experience with skin-to-skin contact. In addition to providing health benefits, touch promotes bonding and social contact. Besides oxytocin, *opioids* (natural morphine-like chemicals) surge within our bodies when we're touched, lowering pain and heightening feel-good sensations. Research shows that parent-child touch brings about the greatest opioid release.[26] Another thing touch does is activate the *orbitofrontal cortex* (a brain structure associated with the processing of emotions), which studies show is linked to depression.[27] So you see, there are many benefits to touch that can help your child experience a boost in well-being. We'll cover just a few of them now.

- *Acupuncture* dates back about five thousand years in China. It is based on the theory that health and wellness depend on a delicate balance of *chi* (energy) and that any blockage along meridian lines where energy flows will cause illness. Eastern medicine believes that each meridian line is associated with an organ or system of the body. Western medicine would define meridian lines as neuron pathways where synapses fire. With acupuncture, a certified acupuncturist inserts ultrathin sterilized needles or uses cutaneous stimulation (a mild electrical current administered on top of the skin) at specific neuron pathways along your child's body. The needles/current free blocked energy, enhancing central nervous system functioning. Acupuncture is safe for children, but only in the hands of a trained practitioner. Pediatric acupuncturists can treat a variety of illnesses and disorders such as ear infections, digestive troubles, respiratory illness, behavioral issues, asthma and allergies, and depression and anxiety.[28] Acupuncture sessions are generally several times a week—and may or may not be covered by medical insurance. According to a study in the journal *Pediatrics*, mild side effects can include a pinching feeling or bruise at the contact site. More serious side effects of infections were rare.[29]
- *Acupressure* is a less invasive method of acupuncture, using pressure by the practitioner's hands or fingers at meridian points. The goal of acupressure is the same as acupuncture—to unblock the flow of energy so healthy synaptic transmission can occur. It's important to note that a child's meridian system is not fully developed until the age of seven or eight, so making sure to work with a pediatric acupressurist is vital. Like acupuncture, acupressure can be useful in the treatment of depression.[30]
- *Exercise* has long been associated with good physical and mental health. Exercise increases oxygen flow to the brain, helps improve cognitive

functioning, sharpens mental skills, decreases stress hormones, and aids in the syntheses of neurotransmitters.[31] With regard to children, regular physical activity has been associated with improved self-esteem, decreased anxiety, and decreased risk for depression.[32] The tricky thing here is that when your child is depressed, or moving into a depression, his body is likely listless, achy, or fatigued—his mood irritable or sullen. Encouraging him to exercise may feel like an impossible feat. When I was depressed as a child, I remember feeling as if I could gather dust because I was so immobilized by the heaviness of my body. I was often splayed out on a couch or a bed, where turning over was an effort in and of itself, never mind the idea of getting up. Encouragement from others ("Maybe if you get out of bed you'll feel better") was always more successful than direct threats ("I'm not gonna keep coming into this room if you don't get out of bed") or hurtful statements ("You're just being lazy. Enough already"). Goals for exercise with a depressed child should aim for short bursts of movement first, like getting up, taking a shower, or walking the dog. Next up might be venturing a little further with an increase in exertion and length of time—a walk around the block or a trip to the store. Model physical activity for your child by exercising as well—whether you do it on your own or with others. Even better is to invite your child to join you in some physical activities such as playing catch, pumping some iron, swatting baseballs, or tending to chores around the house. Once your child experiences moving his body, the opioid release will encourage more feel-good movements into his repertoire.[33] Then activities such as organized sports, organized dance, tai chi, or martial arts can be explored. When it comes to school, physical education teachers and coaches always appreciate it when you make them aware of your child's emotional struggles. This way, disinterest, nonparticipation, or slowed responses can be seen in their real light—as coming from the symptoms of depression, not misbehavior—and can then be handled in supportive ways.

- *Massage therapy* has been used for over three thousand years to heal children and adults. Ancient Egyptians, Persians, Hindus, and Chinese applied forms of massage for many ailments—and Hippocrates wrote papers recommending the use of touch for joint and circulatory problems and physical and emotional illnesses, too. Today, the benefits of massage are varied and far reaching. Massage therapy doesn't only ease stress and relax children—it's also beneficial for many conditions, including anxiety, arthritis, asthma, chronic pain, depression, diabetes, insomnia, and migraines.[34] Massage therapy for children involves various techniques in which muscles and soft tissue are relaxed, toxins are released, *endorphins* flow, and the feel-good hormone oxytocin surges. Incorporating massage into your child's life doesn't necessarily require a professional treatment. You can learn about techniques of massage to add to your child's bedtime routine. Be aware that little ones often welcome your physical gestures, while older teens may squirm at the invitation. If your child shows discomfort with massage, a gentle hug, a stroke of her arm, or a quick squeeze of her hand can still stimulate bonding hormones—and convey a comforting sense of love, security, and trust. There are more than two hundred variations of massage, bodywork, and somatic therapies that can help your child, so make sure to inquire about the style a professional massage therapist uses if you go that route.

- *Showers* are, I think, one of the greatest tools for helping ease depression. When battling depression, if there's only energy to muster one thing, I'd tell you to get your child into the shower. The warmth of the water is soothing and will awaken her skin. See if you can find scented soaps or scrubs to invigorate her muscles and sense of smell, too. If you can, invest in a good showerhead—one that offers different kinds of sprays, pulses, and pressure. I've also recommended a shower stool to help your child sit if she is weak or too fragile to stand. Consider music and flameless candles—and, of course, lots of clean, fluffy towels.

The shower was singularly curative for me as a child—and remains my go-to healing tool even now as an adult. The deadness of my own depression can't fight how the streams of warm water jolt me back to life. Instead of feeling cocooned and constricted, my pores open, blood vessels dilate, and steam floods my lungs and sinuses like puffs of air inflating life back into a balloon. Though it's hard some days to get myself to the shower, I know that once I'm there, I'm golden. And on days that it's easy for me to get into my shower, I use all kinds of aromatherapy to seal the deal.

- *Yoga* is the ancient Indian practice of using poses, stretches, breathing, and visual imagery. Yoga slowly made its way to the Western world in the seventeenth century, and it has exploded in popularity in the last decade as a healing art for children and adults.[35] Like massage, feel-good endorphins are released, while the stress hormone, cortisol, is reduced.[36] Studies show it is excellent at reducing anxiety, heart rate, blood pressure, and respiration for children.[37] Yoga's specific postures, breathing practices, and meditation techniques help your child realign his inner and outer regulatory systems, bringing inner peace as well as improving concentration, body awareness, and mood.[38] The reason I like recommending yoga for a depressed child is that it takes very little to get things going. Yoga can be practiced in a small space, without leaving home, with little gear needed to experience its benefits. On tough days, I've been known to roll out of bed to my yoga mat, where I exercise the breathing, stretching, and core training in my pajamas. Instructional DVDs are available, and your child can do his yoga anytime, anywhere. Maybe you will join him at home with your own mat and make the practice of yoga a bonding experience to share. Classes are available at local gyms and health clubs as well, and schools are even incorporating the remarkable benefits of yoga in classroom curriculum.[39]

Though science suggests moving one's body and the gentle touch of another is an immediate mood lifter, you can add touch to your child's life in other ways. Teach her to really experience different textures and temperatures, like the softness of a cozy blanket, the warmth that comes from feeling sunlight on her skin, or the delicate crush of your lips as you plant a kiss on her cheek.

I've involved myself in all the touch therapies mentioned from childhood through my fifties while growing up with a chiropractor for a father who supplied referrals to specialists who practiced acupuncture, acupressure, reflexology, kinesiology, shinoshin, and reiki—and too many more to name. I've tried all of these touch therapies, and I have discovered that massage therapy provided me with consistent depressive relief—that and yoga, which keeps me feeling fit, balanced, and grounded.

HEARING

Just as research has shown a blunting of other senses with depression, hearing can be affected by it, too. For some children, noises can seem loud and sharp, while for others the sense of hearing is dimmed, almost muffled. Here are some alternative methods for balancing your child's sense of hearing and improving his well-being.

Encourage your child to listen to music. Research shows that music activates the brain's reward system that releases dopamine.[40] Studies also show that listening to music decreases pain, bolsters the immune system, increases feelings of power, and decreases fatigue and depression. It's important, though, to know that different kinds of music can yield different emotional reactions.

There are several musical devices that produce emotional and physical reactions. For example, certain tonal tensions and changes in chords induce physical shivers, prickles on the back of the neck, and a lump in the throat in some people.[41] The musical ornamentation called an *appoggiatura*, a note that clashes with the melody just enough to create a dissonance, can lead to feelings of being overwhelmed, often leaving the listener in tears.[42] Recently Adele's song "Someone Like You" was noted to have many appoggiaturas, explaining why so many people cry when hearing that song. Keep in mind that Yo Yo Ma's cello weeps in the wallows of appoggiaturas, as does a lot of opera. But chances are your child's musical tastes don't lean to the classics. Most likely, your young child is listening to pop or *Billboard* Top 40 songs. Your teenager, though, is more likely to be listening to emotionally charged music, so do consider sharing the research on how listening to such music can worsen mood.

Just before my suicidal attempt as a teenager, I was listening to very melodramatic songs. For me, the music and lyrics conveyed what I was feeling—staggering sadness. The songs that I played over and over on my record player mirrored how alone, lost, and despairing I'd become. At that time in the 1980s, little was known about suicide risks, but nowadays, many parents know that music content can reveal underlying depressive and self-destructive struggles kids are facing.

Research on emotion and music suggests upbeat songs lead to feel-good sensations. Music with power chords, major scales, dynamic chord shifting, and inspirational messages can serve your child well. For me, nothing lifts my spirits like reggae. But just like scents, sounds will be very personal, so let your child choose what works for him.

Another way to invite sound is to suggest audiobooks to your child. There's something so special about the experience of being read to. We loved it as kids, and research shows that audiobooks can be a way for your child to rest and refuel while not feeling alone.[43] Find a book in which the story is an inspiring one or is comical or empowering in content. Audiobooks can be experienced in bed, while sitting on the couch with others or walking, and even on the school bus. And with phones and small computer devices, it's easier than ever to plug into an audiobook.

To help ease the heaviness of depression, consider adding soundscapes to your child's environment. Sometimes called *acoustic sound therapy*, the pleasant background or ambient sounds of birds singing, a soft wind, a babbling brook, or the ocean activate neurons in the cortex, increase dopamine and serotonin production, and increase optimism.[44] You can find soundscapes to purchase on CDs. There are radio stations that exclusively broadcast soundscapes, and there are apps to download onto your child's phone or computer. There are even convenient travel soundscape machines that reproduce soothing sounds, naturescapes, and plain old white noise as well. And remember, an open window provides an instant soundscape so long as it's free from traffic and chaos.

Don't forget the power of your voice as a parent. I don't mean the strength or loudness of it; I mean the significance it carries for your child. When your child hears you speak with love and support, dopamine and oxytocin levels surge. Your voice holds tremendous medicinal powers, so consider whispering encouraging things when you can, leave voicemails for your child, and use the muscle of the pony-express praise by letting you child overhear you praising her or admiring her when you talk with another person.

Once you've helped your child refuel his sense of hearing, teach him to be a good listener.[45] Listening is an art, and it is quite different from hearing. Listening involves not just the mechanics of hearing but also sensing texture, tone, and quality. Listening can enrich the human experience by bringing greater meaning to things heard. So help your child sense the difference in sounds and voices. Cue him into the subtle breathing his kid sister takes when she naps, or the rhythm of his grandpa's laugh, or the rolling feel of a kitten's purr. Teach him to reflect on the sound of his own voice. Is it strong? Does it tremble? What can he learn from it?

One last thought about hearing that I believe doesn't get its rightful due is silence. Though research papers, books, and theories indicate that silence can be a sign of depression, it shouldn't preclude your child from wanting to dwell in its margins. Quietness and stillness are tremendous healing experiences that invite relaxation, improve immune functioning, and self-reflection.[46] Healthy silence has a quietness to its texture and energy, whereas unhealthy silence feels secluded and isolating. When your child wants to have alone time, monitor the quality and quantity of it. It just might be a good thing he's doing. As I kid, I needed a lot of quiet. Without it, the chaos of life crept in and weighed heavily on my already fragile psyche. I've always made time for silence. I still do today. Whether I'm meditating, cat napping, or resting aimlessly on the couch or outside on a chair, I'm replenishing my mind, body, and soul.

THINGS TO REMEMBER

Most traditional methods to treat depression include talk therapy and medication for children and adults. But looking at this complementary approach of feeding the five senses can make it easy to add holistic measures to your child's care. Before this chapter ends, it's important to be mindful of a few things.

1. Remember that depression is an illness of depletion, and it can often result in a dulling of your child's senses.
2. When using holistic measures, research reports success with mild depression. Holistic approaches are generally not recommended solely as a treatment for moderate or severe depression.[47]
3. When working with holistic methods, be an educated consumer and work alongside your pediatrician. Read, research, and find what your child likes and know the ins and outs, the good and the bad, so your expectations can be grounded realistically.
4. Be watchful for *serotonin syndrome*,[48] an increase in serotonin from holistic approaches that can cause concerning side effects. Toxicity can come in mild, moderate, and severe levels, causing agitation, anxiety, and mania. Work in concert with your pediatrician when using holistic methods to prevent this experience.
5. Keep a list of holistic measures your child likes, so if you're away or your child is not home, others can know what will be soothing. Keeping a list at the ready is also a good preventive approach, so if subclinical symptoms present again, you can easily get healing measures going.
6. Remember that recovery is a process. Try not to measure your child's improvement against the experience of another who may be using the same holistic measures.
7. If holistic approaches aren't working, don't view it as a failure. Your child's unique biology may require more traditional approaches to address his or her depression.

The following case study shows how using an alternative treatment for depression can be successful. Remember, though, that holistic methods are recommended for mild cases of depression.

CASE STUDY: REGGIE

Reggie started psychotherapy with me as a middle school student. His mother battled depression herself and noticed similar behaviors in her son "during the school year." I evaluated Reggie's symptoms and behaviors and found that, in fact, Reggie did struggle during the school year—from around November until about March. Furthermore, this was the third winter in which he wrestled getting to school, performing in class, and getting into social skirmishes with his friends. Reggie's depression popped up like clockwork as the days got shorter. And his symptoms slowly disappeared come spring, when the sun lingered longer in the sky. His was a classic case of major depression disorder with a seasonal onset . . . also called seasonal affective disorder.

Reggie's mom was a physical therapist, and she liked using holistic measures in her work and in her personal life. Reggie embraced this lifestyle as much as a young boy could—never really minding his mom's organic meals or healing salves as long as they "didn't smell too bad or taste too bad." Reggie was game for trying out different approaches when illness or injuries presented. So it wasn't a surprise to learn that Reggie and his mom were interested in using bright light therapy along with psychotherapy for his depression. Given that Reggie's seasonal affective onset was mild, I agreed that bright light therapy could be helpful. Together we researched the newest blue light units on the market, and within a few weeks, one arrived in the mail at Reggie's home.

Psychotherapy focused on giving Reggie tools to change his negative thinking, ease his frustrations, be persistent with productive decisions, and keep him on track by not sleeping too much (something that significantly worsened his depression during the winter months). He used bright light therapy every morning to help shift his neurochemistry, and it seemed to greatly keep lift his mood and get him on a healthy sleep schedule. Reggie reported that using bright light therapy was a very easy thing to do. He left it on for fifteen to twenty minutes as he checked into Facebook each morning.

After a few months of teaching Reggie how to deal with his seasonal affective disorder, he appeared happier and more focused—something his mother said never really happened until the summer was in full swing. I recommended that he keep using bright light therapy until the end of the school year, and then measure if the summer sun helped to keep him in good spirits. If so, he was to set the bright light therapy aside to use again once autumn arrived on the calendar. We all agreed that should Reggie's moods decline at any time, he'd return to talk therapy, and if bright light therapy began to NOT offer symptom relief, a change to traditional interventions, such as medication during the winter months, would be considered.

Before treatment ended, I encouraged Reggie to understand the importance of sticking to this regime. Holistic methods, like any intervention, require a long-term commitment—something kids often have trouble maintaining. I also emphasized for Reggie the need to be mindful of this illness and not minimize its magnitude because his depressions would come and go with the seasons. Together with his mother, we helped him understand that this seasonal mood change might remain with him for the rest of his life, and how learning to live successfully with it now would give him a great edge.

It's been three years since I've seen Reggie—three more winters that would challenge his biology and his coping skills. I like to think that all is good there—and that not hearing from his mother means he is managing his seasonal depressions well.

Self-Harm and Suicide

No book on depression would be complete without looking at two serious aspects of depression in children. In this chapter, we will cover self-harm and youth suicide.

Now, I understand how you might be uncomfortable with these topics. No one wants to think these could ever be relevant to his or her child. And then there's the shame and stigma that shrouds these subjects. No matter the reason, it's imperative not only to read this chapter but also to refer to it time and again to make sure your child doesn't resort to these life-threatening behaviors.

The statistics for self-harm and youth suicide are alarming. Self-harm occurs in 15 percent of children and teens[1]—and suicide is the third leading cause of death for children ages ten to twenty-four.[2]

WHAT IS SELF-HARM?

Self-harm is a deliberate behavior in which a child inflicts physical harm on her body to relieve emotional distress. This behavior has a paradoxical effect in that the self-inflicted pain actually sets off an endorphin rush, providing relief. It's important to note that self-injury *does not involve* a conscious intent to commit suicide, and as such, it has been termed *non-suicidal self-injury* (NSSI). This kind of self-injury can take many forms, including cutting, picking, burning, bruising, puncturing, embedding, scratching, or hitting, just to name a few.

In its simplest form, NSSI is a physical solution to an emotional problem. Generally, it's an intentional, private act that is habitual in occurrence, not attention seeking in nature or meant to be manipulative. Children who self-injure are usually secretive about this behavior, rarely letting others know. Girls often cover up their wounds with clothing, bandages, or jewelry. Boys tend to wear long sleeves and long pants—even in the heat of summer.

Symbolically speaking, when a child deliberately injures it's viewed as a method to communicate what cannot be spoken. With self-harm, the skin is the canvas and the cut, burn, or bruise is the paint that illustrates the emotional picture. Most children who self-injure have difficulties with emotional expression. The clinical term for this experience is *alexithymia*, and it is defined as the inability to recognize emotions, their subtleties and textures, and difficulty understanding or describing thoughts and feelings.[3] Many children who self-harm struggle with internal conflicts, usually experiencing depression, anxiety, or other serious psychological concerns such as sexual or physical abuse, eating disorders, or emerging personality disorders. They don't know how to verbalize feelings and, instead, act them out by self-injuring. Studies show girls self-harming more than boys, with onset occurring in childhood. The most concerning fact that research shows is that deliberate, nonsuicidal self-injury can lead to deliberate suicide.[4]

WHEN DEPRESSED KIDS SELF-HARM

The majority of NSSI cases I've seen are depressed children and teens who use cutting as a means of expression—though some children self-harm in other ways (deliberate physical injury resulting in dislocated fingers, broken bones, and embedding items under their skin, just to name a few).

Cuts can take form in delicate lines, swirls, patterns, and initials. Wounds are usually assigned to hidden places, not readily visible to the casual observer. The style and manner of self-harm will be as individual as the child. So, too, will be the instrument chosen. Tools for self-injury can be items specifically designed to cut, such as scissors, knives, and razors. Or ordinary items can be used such as pins, paper clips, pen caps, forks, nail files . . . anything that can break the skin.

Research into self-harm reveals it to be a physiologically and psychologically addictive behavior. Clinical studies link the role of opiates. When a child self-harms, these feel-good endorphins flood the bloodstream. The rush is so pleasing that a child learns to perceive self-harm as soothing, instead of being destructive.[5] This "high" secures a cyclic addiction, making it hard for children to break the cycle of self-harm. *It hurts, but it feels good.* This is similar to *hypnotic analgesia* that wounded soldiers and athletes report experiencing—a high without pain.[6]

WHY IS SELF-HARM SO COMMON?

Media influence is one of the main reasons why self-harm is on the rise. High-profile individuals such as Princess Diana, Johnny Depp, Christina Ricci, Fiona Apple, and Angelina Jolie have revealed that they self-injured. Movies such as *Girl, Interrupted* and *Thirteen* depict children using self-harm as a way to reduce adversity.[7] This gets translated as a possible option for depressed children who may not have more adaptive problem-solving strategies. Another influential factor is peer contagion, when a child learns of other friends who have self-harmed. It suddenly becomes an option not previously considered.[8] A child's inner dialogue may go like this: *If she tried it, maybe this can work for me.*

SELF-HARM INTERVENTIONS

Often, a depressed child who has self-harmed finds his way to me because a friend told a teacher, support staff, or a guidance counselor of the injuries, or a parent notices bloody tissues or marks on his body. However discovered, it is imperative to immediately seek professional mental health help.

The first step is to determine if self-harm is nonsuicidal or suicidal. This will be done with a standard suicide assessment. The clinical inquiry

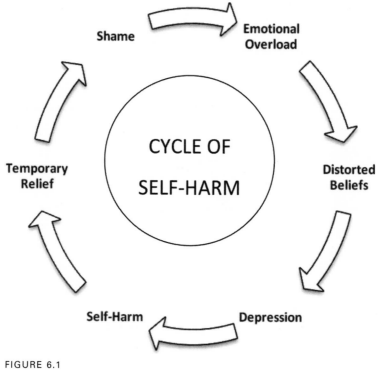

FIGURE 6.1
Cycle of Self-Harm

will address the patterns of self-harm, the conflicts your child is experiencing, as well as mood states before, during, and after injuries.

The second step will help your child understand *the why's* of self-harm. Research shows that children who self-harm are trying to:[9]

- calm overwhelming or unmanageable feelings
- distract themselves from deep sadness
- end feelings of helplessness
- express negative thoughts or feelings that cannot be put into words
- maintain control in chaotic situations
- offset feelings of low self-esteem
- self-nurture or self-care
- self-punish, self-shame, or express self-hate

The last step will help your child put into practice interventions such as *visualization*, using positive imagery to deal with sad or painful experiences; *sensory grounding skills*, learning to use senses to steady oneself, like holding something soft, listening to soothing music, or drawing or writing; and *cognitive grounding skills*, through which your child can learn to ask, "What is really making me sad?" and "What is setting me off?," or to make empowering statements such as "I am safe, and I am in control." These techniques re-orient your child to the here and now, and they can keep the impulse to self-harm from emerging.[10]

FIVE TIPS FOR REDUCING SELF-INJURY IN YOUR CHILD

Once your child has come to understand the cycle of self-harm, it may take a few trials and errors until the behavior is successfully removed. As a parent, here are some ways that you can help your child reduce the urge to self-harm.

1. *Create an emergency kit.* Use a shoe box, plastic zip bag, or other storage container to place positive items to use when an urge hits, things such as photos of friends and family, pictures of idols or heroes, inspiring quotes, uplifting notes, a journal for writing, markers or art supplies for creative expression, a beloved stuffed animal, a CD mix of upbeat music, favorite scents, and other things your child may find soothing.

2. *Use positive imagery.* Help your child strengthen her visualization skills by practicing some yourself. Talk aloud as you describe a beautiful beach scene—or how it feels watching the trees sway in the wind. Conjure up positive memories of places or things you've seen; studies show that describing them in vivid details offers mood-enhancing benefits.[11] Whatever soothing images move you, make sure you *share* and *show* them with your child. Modeling problem-solving strategies in front of your child increases the likelihood she will too.

3. *Point out triggers.* Help your child become aware of the events that weaken his resolve. If it's a test coming up in school, a social event,

or a dentist appointment, talk about how the days leading up to it can feel stressful. Help him learn what kinds of experiences make him sad or irritable. Share what your own triggers are and how you deal with them. Becoming aware of triggers helps your child anticipate negative feelings. Having this advanced warning prevents him from being blindsided emotionally. It allows him to have skills at the ready.

4. *Take a detour.* If your child can't fight the urge, help her reroute self-harm by using less severe activities. For example, holding an ice cube, tearing paper, shredding a sheet, snapping a rubber band, sucking a lemon peel, and pounding a pillow are other ways to diminish the need to self-injure. Suggest the adrenaline rush of running, dancing, holding a yoga pose, jumping rope, or a good game of chase with the family dog to offset urges. The rush of adrenaline from these positive behaviors produces the same chemical surge that comes from self-injury.[12]

5. *Forgive slips.* As your child tries to interrupt self-harming behaviors, know it will not come easily. It's rare that a child, or even an adult for that matter, can stop self-harm cold turkey. There will be days or even weeks when he does well followed by a setback. Should you find that he's lapsed into self-harming, compassionately remind him that change takes time—and that you know he'll find his way again. Offering nonjudgmental support is crucial for recovery. Research shows that shame, criticism, or overreaction when parents see a wound causes children to withdraw back into self-harming behaviors.

SUICIDE IN CHILDREN AND ADOLESCENTS

It's disheartening to read this next sentence. More than four thousand children die by suicide each year. What's more staggering is that it's more than all the deaths of children caused by accidents, wars, and homicides around the world, combined.

Suicide is a significant risk for anyone with a mental illness, but it is exponentially higher for children with depression.[13] As previously mentioned, suicide is the third leading cause of death in children ages ten to twenty-four. But this is only the tip of the iceberg. Every year, approximately 125,000 children are brought to emergency rooms to receive treatment for injuries inflicted from attempting suicide.[14]

WARNING SIGNS AND RISK FACTORS FOR YOUTH SUICIDE

The key to preventing suicide in children is early identification. Two powerful ways to recognize susceptibility in children is by learning warning signs and risk factors. Evidence-based warning signs for youth suicide are presented below.[15] Take a moment and see if your child experiences any of the following:

- anxiety, agitation, sleeping difficulties
- becomes suddenly cheerful after a period of depression
- change in eating habits
- complains of being a bad person or feeling rotten inside
- descending into a depression
- dramatic mood changes
- emerging from an intense depression
- expresses having no reason for living, no sense of purpose
- expressions of wanting or seeking revenge
- feelings of being trapped—like there's no way out
- feelings of hopelessness
- giving or throwing away favorite possessions, cleaning room
- increases alcohol and/or drug use
- loss of interest in fun activities
- not tolerating praise or rewards
- persistent boredom, difficulty concentrating, decline in schoolwork
- preoccupation with songs of death
- rage, uncontrolled anger
- reckless, risky, or running-away behaviors, seemingly without thinking
- statements like "I won't be a problem for you much longer," "Nothing matters," and "It's no use."
- unusual neglect of personal appearance
- withdrawal from friends, family, and regular activities

While warning signs are behaviors that alert a child may be suicidal, risk factors are biochemical, psychological, and social experiences that increase the likelihood of suicide.[16] Take a look and see if any relate to your child:

- abuse, sexual or physical
- access to alcohol and drugs
- access to lethal weapons
- biochemical vulnerabilities
- breakup in a romantic relationship
- cultural beliefs supporting suicide
- diagnosis of depression or bipolar disorder
- financial hardships
- GLBT sexual orientation
- having a familial history of suicide
- loss of a parent due to death, divorce, or separation
- media reports of suicide
- medication akinesia
- previous suicide attempt
- problem with the law
- rapid sociocultural changes
- recent loss of a friend or family member
- school failure
- stressful life events
- unplanned pregnancy
- untreated mental illness
- victim of bullying

There were plenty of warning signs and risk factors back when I was a teenager before I attempted suicide. First was that I was already struggling for years with an untreated mental illness, dysthymic disorder. That set the stage for being vulnerable to the life events I was facing. One of them was college, which was challenging because I had to achieve high grades in order to keep my academic scholarship. I was a commuter student, and

I found it difficult to break into social groups or find friends on campus. I was very lonely and disconnected socially. My home life was chaotic, with my parents fighting frequently. And I had also experienced a sexual assault, which left me feeling despair and great shame. My downward spiral continued with feelings so overwhelming in their breadth and depth that I lost track of time. My judgment became muddled, my thinking grew negative, and my sense of hope crumbled. Within weeks of falling into a major depressive episode, I was planning to die by suicide.

It's easy, now, to see the decline in my mental, emotional, and physical states, but back then, I had no idea I was ill. Neither did anyone else. The culture wasn't tuned into suicide prevention or detection back then. And it is truly by sheer luck that I am alive today.

Depression robs children of their sensibilities—which are delicate and vulnerable to begin with. When severe, the neurobiology of depression twists thinking, often leaving little or no room for hope. From my clinical perspective, that's the most dangerous thing about depression—when thinking gets deformed. From my personal perspective, my flat and fixed thinking led me down a lethal, one-way road. My teenage depressed mind believed that suicide was a practical solution.

It's important for you, as a parent, to understand how depression infects the clarity of your child's mind like a virus attacks the body. What makes sense to you will not make sense to your child. The words *options* or *choices* won't be appreciated, nor will the phrase "things will get better, you'll see." When the grip of depression tightens its hold, you must do everything you can to help your child conquer it.

UNDERSTANDING SUICIDALITY

This next section looks at the kinds of suicide behaviors children display. It may be tough to read, even more difficult to imagine, but learning about the different levels of *suicidality* can help you intervene quickly to help your child.

Clinically speaking, suicidality is defined as a series of ideas and behaviors, ranging from subconscious thoughts to the act of suicide itself.

Researchers specializing in diagnosing and treating suicide believe that detailing distinct categories of suicidality helps identify at-risk children, as well as aids in prevention and intervention efforts.[17]

1. *Self-harm behavior with subconscious suicidal intent* is the category that describes the actions of children who hurt, wound, or harm themselves without understanding the intentions of their behavior. This is different from nonsuicidal self-injury (NSSI) mentioned above. This is when self-harm moves into intentional harm. Often, the self-harm act has a careless or ambiguous tone of its own. *I totally don't know how I cut my wrist. I'm not sure how I swallowed so many pills. The car came out of nowhere and hit me as I crossed the street.* Inquiring further about "unintended" cuts or wounds, self-destructive behaviors, or "accidental" overdosing may reveal feelings of unworthiness, guilt, and despair, and pessimistic attitudes in children.

2. *Suicidal ideation,* sometimes called "suicidal thinking," is the stage in which a child consciously thinks about suicide. The thoughts of sleeping forever, not waking up, or being dead fall in this category, as do more detailed fantasies about how death by suicide could happen.

3. *Suicidal intent* is the category in which thought is accompanied by the intention to perform the suicidal act. For some children, intent is expressed but with no active plan to carry it out. *I think I could find my dad's gun, but I wouldn't really use it.* Others, though, express intent to act on their suicidal urges and express a specific manner in which they intend to carry out their intentions. *I'm gonna wait 'til everyone's asleep and use my dad's gun.*

4. *Preparatory acts toward imminent suicide* is the category in which suicidal ideation and intent move into full-on action. A number of children start taking care of personal issues, such as giving things away, throwing items out, cleaning their room, or asking siblings or friends to take care of things for them. Sometimes children vocalize their preparation with phrases like "I won't be around much longer to see this," or "Things will be easier when I'm not around." This is the stage

when the suicide plan becomes actualized and the items or methods for suicide are sought out and stored away for use, such as pills, firearms, a rope, or a knife.

5. *Interrupted suicide attempt* is the category in which a child initiates a death by suicide but is interrupted by another person, an outside circumstance, or by their own self-reflection. No physical harm or injury occurs in this category, although the emotional toll of the experience can wither a child to an even more fragile state.

6. *Nonfatal suicide attempt* is the category that describes a suicide attempt that was carried out by a child but was not fatal. Perhaps the overdose wasn't toxic enough, the rope frayed and broke apart, the cut wasn't lethal, or the gun misfired. I have worked with many children who've had nonfatal suicide attempts.

7. *Completed suicide* is the category describing a death by suicide.

By the time I was acting out my plan to die by suicide, I had already passed through several levels of suicidality. Thirty years ago, no one talked openly about the steps leading up to suicide. Prevention wasn't like it is nowadays. Perhaps if I knew back then about the degrees of suicidality, I might have sought help. Maybe my parents would've noticed more. I bet even my friends would've sensed something was terribly wrong with me. But that's not how it happened. It is by sheer luck that I am here, alive, today.

Some parents make the mistake of thinking the early stages of suicidality are not serious enough to seek immediate help. *It's all just talk.*

I can't tell you how many times I've heard a parent say that phrase. Sometimes it comes from denial. Sometimes it stems from ignorance. My reflex is to advise every parent to seek intervention the second any of these behaviors appear.

THE IMPORTANCE OF A SUICIDE PREVENTION PLAN

One way inoculate your child from falling into the depths of a suicidal despair is to put together a suicide prevention plan. I encourage you and your child to create this plan together—bringing integrity, dignity, and hope into the experience, and not fear, shame, or worry. The message to your child will be "This is what we are going to do to keep you safe."

1. *Have an "action plan."* Keep a list of doctors, professionals, agencies, and hotlines near all landline telephones. These should also be programmed into all mobile and cordless phones and bookmarked in personal computers and laptops.

2. *Sequester lethal means.* Consider putting prescriptions and over-the-counter medications under lock and key. Keep items such as razors, knives, firearms, rope, and other lethal items out of reach by locking them up, throwing them out, or having someone safeguard them.

3. *Remove drugs and alcohol.* Substance use increases impulsivity and blurs problem-solving skills. Keep all alcohol and drugs out of reach by locking them up or throwing them away.

4. *Involve your child's school support staff.* Make sure you bring school personnel on board so they can support your child during the school day. Psychologists, counselors, and social workers can create a nurturing space to talk, rest, or refuel. Doing so helps prevent depressive symptoms from worsening and ensures greater communication should the grip of suicidal thinking occur at school.

5. *Ask the tough questions.* Don't be afraid to ask your child if he's thinking about hurting himself or is having thoughts about dying by suicide. Research has shown that asking *will not* increase a child's risk. Rather, studies have shown children are often relieved to talk about it. Your concerns as a parent and the love your feel in your heart helps counter your child's hopelessness and helplessness.

6. *Be prepared to act.* If you detect your child's judgment and thinking have deteriorated, immediately contact a health care professional. If you cannot wait, take your child to the nearest hospital emergency room yourself—or call a friend or family member to help. If your child resists, don't be afraid to call the police. They are trained to deal with

such matters. My experiences having the police come to my office to escort a family to the hospital have been positive each and every time.

WHAT TO EXPECT SHOULD YOUR CHILD NEED HOSPITALIZATION

Not every child who is depressed will have suicidal thoughts or feelings. But of those who do, sometimes going to the hospital is necessary. In my practice, I like to educate parents about what to expect when hospitalization occurs.

For starters, it's not straitjackets, rubber rooms, and metal beds. Those images are inaccurate and stigmatizing. Child and adolescent inpatient programs are generally housed within a hospital, but they are arranged like college dormitories. The unit itself has single, double, or triple rooms for sleeping, and common areas for relaxing. It is a locked and secured environment. This is to keep your child and others safe, and it enables the team staff, which is present throughout the day and night, to manage everyone on the floor with continuity. The team of professionals will likely include psychiatrists, psychologists, social workers, nurses, nutritionists, recreational therapists, art therapists, schoolteachers, and pediatricians.

Once there, your child will be evaluated for admission to the unit by a crisis team and assigned a clinician case worker. For safety purposes, there will be rules regarding acceptable clothing, accessories, and food. During the week, your child will follow a schedule, with meals, classes, treatments, and recreation—much like the kind of schedules found in schools. Weekends have less structure, and the staff will make allowances for more recreation or home passes off the unit when goals are reached.

It's important to note that your child may bear witness to children who have struggles similar to, less than, or more intense than her own. Though it may be distressing at first, over time it can show her how other children work to conquer their own issues.

As a parent, your participation will be extremely valuable. No one knows your child better than you—and inpatient hospital programs count on your input. It is also expected that you'll attend family sessions when they are requested, and visit your child on a regular basis. Usually, anyone can come and visit your child as long as they are on a list you provide. There are visiting hours every day in most child and adolescent units. Pay phones are also available to talk and check in with your child, usually operational during set hours, such as 5 p.m. to 9 p.m., for example.

The average hospital stay for a child is one week,[18] although your child may stay less or more, depending of the severity of symptoms. The goal of the inpatient program is to decrease the intensity of depression, decrease the risk for suicide, improve coping skills, and achieve other measurable goals determined at the intake. When they are reached, your child will be discharged—with a return to treatment with her outside therapist, with whom the team will have been in contact with during your child's stay.

Inpatient hospitalization may upset or frighten you—or make you worry that you will be judged or criticized because your child cannot cope with her depression. These feelings are not uncommon. Remember, depression isn't a result of poor parenting or laziness. And suicidal thinking doesn't happen to kids because they're weak or not smart enough to know how to fix things. Depression is a serious illness that has numerous causes. Professionals at the inpatient program know this—and they know how hard it was to make this decision.

Hospitalizing your child takes grit and courage, and don't ever let anyone tell you otherwise. As you will see in the following case study, every parent who journeys down this road is a guardian of love and hope.

CASE STUDY: MARK

Mark kicked the end table, sending it to the floor. It was wicker, so it wasn't heavy, but seeing this sixth-grade boy throw a fit of rage within seconds of meeting me left me breathless.

"I don't wanna be here!" he shouted as it fell on the ground.

"Well, you don't have to stay," I said calmly, opening the door to the waiting room. "If you want to leave, you can, Mark."

Mark's father, Jeff, bolted up from his seat, ready to yell at his son. Instead, he gritted his teeth and spoke calmly. "Remember, you can't go back to school if you don't see the doctor."

"Fine!" Mark shouted, and stomped to the couch and sat down.

The oldest of three children, Mark lived with his parents, Jeff and Lynn, until age ten—and then his world fell apart. Jeff described his marriage as "empty but for the kids," and said that he and Lynn separated amicably about four months ago. The children were very traumatized by the split, possibly because, Jeff said, he and his wife never fought. Mark and his sisters stayed at home with their mother, while Jeff found an apartment in town. Jeff reported that both he and Lynn worked hard to co-parent consistently and were in couples therapy to decide whether to divorce or rebuild the marriage. Family history was remarkable for mental illness, as anxiety and mood disorders were prevalent in both family trees—as was alcoholism.

Mark was suspended from school for throwing a chair at his teacher earlier in the week—and he wasn't allowed back until he was seen by a psychologist. Recently, at home, he was found sneaking alcohol and cough medicine. And at his father's apartment, he kicked a hole in the wall after refusing to make his bed. Before his anger erupted, Mark was sullen and depressed and performing poorly in school.

Mark was tall and thin, seeming much older than his age. He had angular features, kept his hair on the long side, and fixed a scowl across his face. Over the next few sessions, I came to learn that he was angry at the world. He was angry at change. He *hated rules* and *hated life*. I believed that Mark was grieving over his parents' separation, but complicating things was his use of alcohol and over-the-counter drugs to cope with stress. He was oppositional. He was defiant. He was also very depressed.

During the next session, we formed a connection, but it was challenging. Mark was direct with his words, but he was not very reflective in his thinking. He seemed impulsive, too, quick to get physical if he was angry, pounding the seat cushions, flipping the chessboard, and launching tissue boxes into the air. I noticed that these actions were never close enough to hurt me, and I came to learn that his chair-throwing episode in school had a similar style. Mark expressed that he'd never want to hurt anyone, but sometimes he got so angry that he couldn't take it anymore. When he threw things, it made him feel better. When he punched a hole in a wall, or kicked in the furniture, it made him feel better. He admitted that even though his hand hurt and his foot throbbed, that it didn't matter to him—because he always felt better afterward.

I suggested to Mark that maybe he was using self-harm as well as drugs and alcohol to shift his irritable and depressed mood states. He didn't agree, but he didn't disagree either. He did, however, complain that he didn't like that the alcohol was moved at his mother's and father's houses—and that the cough medicine "disappeared."

At the third session, Mark expressed his displeasure at not being able to get high and that he hated how he was feeling. He said he hadn't broken anything in the past week, but instead of feeling proud about that, he reported feeling worse. Without the drugs and alcohol— and the use of self-harm—Mark's emotional conflicts took center stage. And they were overwhelming him.

Mark expressed how he didn't want to live anymore—that it would be easier for everyone if he wasn't around. When I asked him to tell me more about these thoughts, Mark revealed how he was spending a lot of time out by the railroad tracks, putting quarters on the rails so the trains would flatten them. He liked how hot and smooth they felt. He told me that sometimes he wanted to lie down on the tracks and "let the train come." When pressed further, Mark explained how he'd just do it, like when he punches a wall.

And then he said, "Almost did it yesterday."

Luckily, Mark's descent into suicidal thinking was observable. Some children don't show their pain or their intent, which raises the likelihood of suicide. This is always the scariest part of depression—when a child's thinking gets distorted. When sound judgment evaporates. When problem solving moves from productive to destructive.

I immediately coordinated an inpatient hospitalization, finding a bed at the child annex for Mark. Together with his parents, we explained how this was a necessary step needed to keep him safe. Mark screamed and yelled, this time cursing at me, telling how he'd never, ever, talk to me again. I told him I understood that he was mad, but that I'd rather he be alive and angry than not here at all.

Though Mark protested about going, he didn't put up a fight when it was time to leave my office. Mark remained at the treatment hospital for almost two weeks. During his stay, I called him each week during common hour, and he told me how things were going and that it wasn't so bad being there. I also remained in contact with Lynn and Jeff, who said the daily therapy, group sessions, and family work were really helping.

Upon discharge, Mark made the decision to work with another therapist he met at the hospital. His mother, Lynn, told me that he was worried that I'd be upset or offended. Of course, I wasn't. I spoke to Mark and let him know that getting better and feeling stronger was all that mattered.

Some of the most wonderful moments happen not when I'm in my office, but when I'm out shopping or running an errand. I feel a hand touch my shoulder or catch the pull of a person's gaze.

"Dr. Deb? I thought that was you!" Lynn said.

It took me a moment to place the face and register the connection. "Oh my god, how are you? How's Mark?

"He's a lawyer now."

A broad smile spread across my face. "That's so great."

"And he just got engaged."

"Wow," I replied.

For the next few minutes, we lingered in the aisle of the store, with Lynn telling me how things played out with her and Jeff. How the kids found their way through it all, and how Mark's hospitalization was the hardest, but most meaningful experience.

Decisions to hospitalize are never easy, and it can bring about extreme reactions in children as well as parents. But in my professional experience working with depressed children, the outcomes have always been positive. In fact, they are often *the* life-changing moment that sets a new trajectory.

7

My Child Is Diagnosed, Now What?

Now that you've learned how pediatric depression is diagnosed and what treatments are recommended, let's detail more about what comes next. In this chapter, you'll understand just what psychotherapy will and won't do for your child—and what you, as a parent, need to do to make treatment successful. The truth about medication for child depression will be presented as well, and ways to deal with stigma will be explored. My goal for this chapter is that you will develop realistic expectations for treatment and are able to separate fact from sensational fiction.

WHAT TO EXPECT FROM PSYCHOTHERAPY

1. *Psychotherapy cannot be successful unless your child wants to be there.* Studies show that forcing your child into psychotherapy is never a good idea.[1] It's true that talk therapy will reduce depressive symptoms, but your child may not agree. Some kids view psychotherapy as "boring," "stupid," and "pointless"—or feel the smack of stigma that wrongly portrays talk therapy being only for "crazy" or "demented" people. Sometimes children feel trapped into coming for an appointment. Out of concern and love, parents force children and teens into therapy before they are ready. The problem is this: If your child feels coerced into going to therapy, the helplessness from depression

worsens. Children can feel resentful, angry, and certain that no one is truly hearing them. It's important to know that a therapist might rework the session to give the decision-making power back to the child if coercion is detected. This is not done to challenge your role as the parent, but to give your child the control and choice needed for therapy to work.

2. *Psychotherapy will not fix your child. Your child will fix himself.* The job of a psychotherapist is *to help your child help himself.* Think of the Chinese proverb: "Give a man a fish; you feed him for a day. Teach a man to fish; you feed him for a lifetime." In therapy, your child will learn how to use skills to kick depression to the curb. Through self-awareness, your child will develop ways to detect triggers, shift negative thinking styles, and manage mood fluctuations. The goal of psychotherapy is not advice giving—in which the child becomes dependent on the therapist to "tell him how to solve this." The purpose of talk therapy is to create skill building, through which your child resolves how to use the techniques, when to use them, where to use them, and which ones work best. From this unique experience come resiliency and independence.

3. *Psychotherapy may not always make your child feel better.* When children make the decision to go to therapy, most of the time it will be a fun and enjoyable experience. Children enjoy having this special time, when their thoughts, interests, and feelings take center stage. There are, however, times when sessions may rub up against a delicate subject, making your child irritable or even upset. Growth involves risks and shifts, as well as facing difficult thoughts and feelings. All of this can be scary for children. Mental health therapists are trained to expect these moments and know how to help children move through them. It's valuable for you to know that the journey can sometimes be bumpy.

4. *Psychotherapy will not work if you have unrealistic expectations.* Make sure you and your child's therapist schedule time to talk about treatment goals. This discussion should also include what realistic expectations to hold. Studies show that the more grounded your hopes are for therapy, the more successful treatment will be for your child.[2] Remem-

ber, therapy has a different time, cadence, and rhythm for each child. This happens because children adapt and grow at different rates. Try not to measure how another child is progressing in therapy in contrast to your own child. When you set your expectations realistically, you'll respond appropriately to your child's progress and be sensitive and accepting if setbacks occur.

5. *Psychotherapy requires your child to be comfortable with your therapist.* One of the most important elements in therapy is for your child to be comfortable with her therapist. There's a lot of chemistry needed for this relationship to "click"—or, in clinical terms, to have a "working alliance." Without this connection, it will be difficult for your child to feel relaxed enough to face difficult issues, feel safe to reveal herself, let go of fears, or try out new behaviors. It's also important that you feel connected to the therapist as well. If not, your child may pick up on your reluctance or dislike, which can have negative effects on treatment. If you or your child doesn't find this compatible connection, don't hesitate to seek out another professional. Finding a "good fit" in therapy is more important than in *any other kind* of professional relationship your child will ever have in his life.

WHAT PARENTS CAN DO TO HELP PSYCHOTHERAPY

It's been long known that a parent's positive attitude toward an experience greatly motivates a child.[3] So keeping a supportive stance on psychotherapy can bolster your child's optimism for depression recovery. Whenever possible, talk confidently about psychotherapy—the meaningfulness of the treatment, the changes noted, the courage your child has shown, the progress made. Avoid openly complaining of the challenges psychotherapy sometimes presents (the time it takes to drive to the appointment, the weekly commitment, the cost, the time you spend waiting in the reception room, etc.). Make sure you keep all appointments and arrive timely for sessions. This makes psychotherapy a consistent intervention in her life, as well as teaching dedication and commitment. It also shows her that in order to deal effectively with depression, one has to continually work at it.

If your child is resistant in going to therapy, lead by example. Consider making an appointment for yourself, alone, to learn how to work on things. Share when your appointment is, what your therapist is like, and talk about the experience when it fits smoothly into conversations. This allows her to see that the process is not a negative one—and that there's no shame in seeking help. All of these actions repeatedly educate and encourage your child to consider taking part in the process as well. If stigma finds its way into your child's world, consider re-educating whoever is spouting misinformation. Help others understand that words such as *crazy, psycho,* and *wacko* perpetuate shameful notions of mental illness. Advocate for your child by supporting news, stories, or research that portrays depression accurately and honestly. Show her the hundreds of famous people in appendix B who have lived with depression and have done amazing things *not in spite of it,* but perhaps *because of it.*

WHAT TO EXPECT FROM MEDICATION

1. *Medication won't work unless you support its use in your child's treatment.* For some depressed children, the need for antidepressant medication will be a vital part of their recovery. Research shows, however, that public opinion about antidepressants is not consistent with scientific knowledge and clinical experience.[4] Many wrongly believe that antidepressants are addictive, change a child's personality, or become a "crutch" if prescribed. These myths not only misinform but can also prevent children from reaching levels of well-being because parents fear their use. If your child needs antidepressant medication, it's strongly recommended that you understand the neurobiology of depression and how antidepressants work. Just like promoting a positive attitude about psychotherapy, parents need to endorse the use of medication so children will be confident taking them.[5]

2. *Medication can only be successful if your child takes it consistently and "as prescribed."* One of the biggest causes of *relapse* of child depression is not being consistent with medication.[6] As a parent, help your child learn the name of the medicine prescribed, the regular time of day or

night it's to be taken, whether it should be given with food, and when the refill date is so no gap in treatment occurs. It's important to understand that missing doses interrupts the effectiveness of medicine, which in turn will get in the way of therapeutic success. Also vital is learning how to use over-the-counter medications if your child is on antidepressant medication. Checking with your pharmacist, psychiatrist, or physician whenever using additional medicines can help avoid *serotonin syndrome*, in which too much serotonin arises in the body.[7] For example, when taking SSRIs, a regular child dose of cough medicine might need to be halved. Along this line is also the significance of educating children not to use alcohol or drugs so substances don't interfere with, or raise toxic levels of, antidepressant medication.

3. *Medication can have side effects, but rarely are they serious.* Any medicine your child takes poses side effects. From aspirin to cough medicine or antibiotics to vitamins—and antidepressants can have side effects, too. Research shows that most children experience mild or moderate levels of side effects and that adjustments in dosage or timing can help manage them. While this is generally the rule, parents should also know that there are many children who don't report any side effects whatsoever. But it's the data on serious side effects that, though rare, make antidepressant treatment a scary subject. For some children, the side effects from taking medication outweigh the benefits. In this case, medication should be stopped, as no one should endure headaches, diarrhea, or stomachaches if they're intense and don't go away with dosage management. There are also emotional side effects, the kinds that leave children feeling dulled or different, which makes it hard for them to want to continue antidepressant treatment.[8] Then there is the rare side effect syndrome called *akinesia*, in which extreme restlessness and agitation heighten violence toward the self or others. This is what the FDA "black box" label warning is about—raising awareness to consumers that antidepressants may increase the risk of suicidal thinking and behavior in some children and adolescents with depression.[9] These are very real issues and require your attention as a parent.

4. *A child or teen taking antidepressant medication should never stop it abruptly.* Once started, treatment with these medications should not be stopped without working with a medical doctor. Although they are not habit-forming or addictive, suddenly ending an antidepressant can cause a withdrawal-like experience called *antidepressant discontinuation syndrome* (a temporary event in which your child might have flulike symptoms). Hastily stopping medication can also lead to relapse or recurrence of depression.[10] If you or your child wants to end antidepressant treatment or wishes to have a scheduled break from it, work with your prescribing doctor to do it appropriately. Often, the weaning period is finished within just a few weeks, without any health concerns.

5. *For some children, taking medication long term to manage depression may be a necessity.* By and large, the course of taking antidepressants is one year. The treatment starts off with a low dose for children, with an expected six to eight weeks for medicine to reach its full effects.[11] From there, the months that follow allow medicine to slowly shift neurochemistry. Working in concert with medication is talk therapy, and the collaboration helps to reduce depressive symptoms and build skills. Once goals are reached, your child can come off medication. But should depressive symptoms present again, chronic use of medication may be necessary. The likelihood of you being faced with this issue is great, as studies show that upward of 40 percent of children with depression will have recurrences.[12] For some parents, the choice to continue medication will be easy, while for others it'll be tough. The truth is making decisions about medication is part science, part emotion. So remember to listen to your heart but take your brain with you.

WHAT PARENTS CAN DO TO HELP WITH MEDICATION

I understand the anxiety that comes with thinking about medication for your child. Before I began antidepressant treatment for my depression I worried about side effects and long-term use. I also held my breath wondering what I'd do *if the medicine didn't work.* At that time, I was an adult as well as a practicing clinician. Knowing that even I had doubts should give you all the permission you need to feel entitled to your worries.

One of the best ways to ease the concerns about side effects is to get into the habit of recording your child's overall well-being. I strongly recommend using side-effect checklists *before* and *during* medication use like the ones in appendix A.

Documenting your child's physical and emotional state before medication is called a *baseline*. As time goes by with your child on antidepressants, record another series of the side-effect checklist. Once you have this data, you can truly measure if side effects are greater as a result of medication use.

As with talk therapy, children may improve at different rates with medication, so be mindful about how you measure your own child's improvements. Whenever possible, talk confidently about medication and lead by example by making sure you follow directions, dosaging, and refilling on time with your own prescriptions.

One of the biggest wedges in pharmacotherapy is when children resist taking medication. Sometimes it's because they don't like the taste of the pill. If so, ask your child's prescribing doctor if the medication comes in liquid form. Refusal to take medicine can be a controlling tactic for children. Often, a child with an illness feels helpless and small, so huffing and puffing about blowing the pill house down is a common occurrence. Try to reason with your child about how taking medicine will help her feel better and that it isn't a sign of weakness or that she's damaged. Taking medicine is just like needing eyeglasses to read or braces to align teeth. It helps makes things better. Never punish your child for not taking medication if he outwardly refuses to do so—or shame him in any way. It's best to express your disappointment and hope that he'll reconsider. Just like forcing a child to therapy, forcing a child to take medicine makes you the bad guy. If he's busy being angry at you for making him do things, he never looks inward to understand how to live with his depression.

Finally, with regard to the stigma of medication, studies show that children who feel shame about medication often struggle socially.[13] To build confidence, be sure that you convey medication in a positive light. It's also recommended for you and your child to disclose *selectively* to others about his medication—the kinds of individuals who'll likely support its use. The approach is suggested not to offset shame regarding antidepressant treatment. Actually, it is just the opposite—it's about safeguarding confidence in a world that still misunderstands mental illness.

As you read the following case study, see how the use of the side-effect checklists and an approach of letting a child make decisions about medication made for a deeper commitment to treatment.

CASE STUDY: TREVOR

Trevor, a tense yet spirited twelve-year-old boy, came in for therapy to deal with his oppositional stance in taking medication. For several years he readily took an SSRI to help his obsessive compulsive disorder, but he had been fighting to avoid taking it.

I met with his parents, Rita and David, who described previous behavioral therapy and medication as "miracles" for helping Trevor reduce his worries, obsessions, and repetitive behaviors. But since moving into middle school, Trevor started resisting taking his medicine.

"First he said he didn't like the side effects," Rita said.

"Then he talked about wanting to fly solo—without it," David replied.

Trevor's parents reported that he never complained about side effects before or appeared uncomfortable with taking medication. They shared how they sometimes bribed him each morning to take it (extra computer time) or punished him when he refused (taking away his cell phone for the day). Trevor's parents were confused as to why he wanted to risk the return of feeling worried and anxious, and they were concerned that his on-and-off-again use of medication could lead to a recurrence. Furthermore, his parents stated that if he wasn't moping around the house when they made him take his medications, he was crying in his room. He appeared to be more sullen and sad, with negative obsessions slowly taking hold again.

I explained to Rita and David that it wasn't unusual to see children distancing themselves from medication, especially at Trevor's age. Psychologically speaking, the pull of independence takes some kids to this point. They want to see if they can work out their issues on their own—without medicine. Another reason may be the urge just to challenge authority, so it's a way of testing limits. Medically, growth spurts and body changes shift metabolism rates, which can truly make for icky side effects where once there were none. So, there was that possibility, too.

"Any or all of these examples could be going on," I said to Trevor's parents.

I encouraged Trevor and his parents to consider the following arrangement: a break from medication to test the waters. As expected, Trevor was all smiles, while a look of disbelief swept across his parents' faces. Together with his prescribing doctor, Trevor would be weaned off the medication and then a scheduled break would unfold. While he was off medicine, he and his parents would fill out symptom side-effect checklists. This would serve as his baseline should he go back on medicine. They'd also note how Trevor was doing at school by touching base with his teachers.

Arranging this break allowed Trevor to feel in control. It also let him see if he could manage his obsessions and his worries with the skills learned in therapy *without the addition of medication*. Gone would be the tug-of-war over taking medication.

Two months later, Trevor returned for a check-in appointment. He told me how he came off his medications and how no more fighting was going on at home. But as much as he wanted to be able to keep his anxieties and circular worries from returning, they crept back in. Trevor told me how he hated these worries more than anything else. "Even more than taking medicine," he said.

Trevor decided to go back on his previous SSRI medication—a decision he made on his own. That very night, his parents picked up his low-dose prescription, and the next day, Trevor took his medication without hesitation. After several weeks, he and his parents completed another side-effect checklist. Using both measures, we saw that Trevor wasn't experiencing any significant side-effect setbacks. His grades improved, his OCD symptoms reduced, his depressive symptoms were gone, and his home and social life were without conflict. Showing Trevor these facts helped put his feelings about returning to take medicine into a more realistic perspective. After a few more weeks, Trevor reported "feeling good," though he felt "sad" that he couldn't keep his obsessions and worries from popping up without medicine.

I took that moment in his session to share with him how I, too, sometimes felt *disappointed* that I had to take medicine.

"For what?" he asked.

"For depression," I replied. "I tried to use my skills, just like you did, to keep me from feeling sad and upset, but I learned that I couldn't do it on my own."

Trevor fell quiet.

"I need the medicine. Just like you," I said.

"Wow, really?"

"Yup, really," I replied.

I spent the rest of the session helping Trevor understand the differences between sadness, disappointment, and grief—some of the many textured experiences people feel about needing to take medicine. We talked about how it was hard to share with friends about things like depression or OCD. But I did not just want him to feel safe enough to explore those thoughts and emotions—I wished for him to not be ashamed about needing medicine in his life.

It's something Trevor is still working on. And I'll get him there.

8

Tips for Parenting
Your Depressed Child

Being a parent fills you with joys and heartaches and millions of in-between moments that make for precious memories. From baby to toddler and all the way through adolescence, you'll be overwhelmed, amazed, delighted, and distressed. The main goal of good parenting is to help your child grow into a healthy adult. To have the necessary skills for life's challenges. To be happy and secure. To love well and find purpose and meaning in life. Although parenting a depressed child can be challenging, there are ways to make these dreams a reality.

CREATING A SUPPORTIVE HOME BASE

Studies show that creating an open and supportive home for your child deepens security and allows your child to feel less ashamed of her mental illness.[1] This means crafting a healthy environment in both the way your home is set up to the way you and family members talk and relate.

Your child's home should be a place she feels physically comfortable, with at least one space, like her bedroom, where she's cozy. Adding to the sense of physical security at home is the use of touch. Don't hesitate to hug, pat, high five, or cuddle if permission is granted. As previously mentioned in chapter 5, touch increases the feel-good hormone oxytocin and reduces the unpleasant stress hormone cortisol.

Emotionally speaking, make sure you work to keep communication open, allowing her to come to you without judgment in order to share her feelings, doubts, or worries. Your child may also display anger, self-pity, and bitterness about the way depression grips her life. Let her express her disappointment, but don't let her wallow too long in it. With young children who are depressed, talking may not be their strong suit. Instead, creative arts such as coloring or drawing can help them communicate struggles to you. So keep an abundance of crayons, colored pencils, and paper around. Though some older children and teens are verbally expressive, don't be surprised if texting or emails are how they reach out to you. Whatever way the communication arrives, always try to talk in person when time allows. Let your child know she can always count on your physical presence.

Having a child with an illness places pressure not only on you as a parent but also on siblings. Sometimes brothers or sisters feel jealous that your depressed child may get more of your attention. Siblings can feel lonely, too—and even worry that they might "catch" depression. Make sure you spend time with your other children—and let your depressed child know that everyone in the family needs special time together. Whenever possible, the home should be a place where talking about depression is welcomed. Though jokes and lighthearted teasing happen among siblings, make sure family members never cross the line into shameful name-calling or degrading phrases. Medication, if used, should be stored in a safe place—away from prying eyes, but not too secluded. Otherwise, this sends a message that it's embarrassing to have such medicine around. And as for scheduled appointments, make sure they're listed on a calendar, both so you know the date and time and so your child sees it, too.

CREATING A SUPPORTIVE SCHOOL BASE

It's often a good idea to reach out to your child's school, especially his teacher(s). Research tells us that pediatric depression is significantly associated with school and social difficulties.[2] By forming a relationship with the school, support services can be created to ease academic or interpersonal pressures. Staff members such as a guidance counselor, nurses, social workers, or psychologists can provide a safe place to go if symptoms arise. This supportive arrangement fosters a sense of belonging for your child, which will deepen his self-identity, positive adjustment, and trust of others. Furthermore, studies show that when a child finds school a protective and caring place, he's less likely to become involved in substance or alcohol abuse—serious risk factors associated with depression.[3] Another benefit of a supportive school base will help your child build resilience. When teachers know a child is struggling with depression, it allows them to challenge and encourage them in more therapeutic ways. If your child fails a test or experiences academic problems, teachers can help him view these as minor obstacles and not personal failures—helping to break the pattern of negative thinking.

Informing the school about your child's depressive disorder can also keep him safe. By design, schools are well equipped to recognize depression, especially with regard to self-harm and suicidal thinking. Staff members are trained and experienced in identifying warning signs for children at risk.[4] Should a crisis occur at school, you can feel assured that a swift and professional response will occur.

While some depressed children may require these minimal supportive interventions, others may not need assistance during the school day at all. The severity of your child's depression and his coping styles will determine what he'll need. If, however, your child is struggling extensively in school, psychoeducational testing can be done to see if he meets the criteria for special education services under the Individuals with Disabilities Education Act. Should a learning disability be discovered, accommodations such as a smaller class setting or extra time on tests can be arranged.[5]

DISCIPLINE YOUR DEPRESSED CHILD

Discipline comes from the word *disciple*, which, in Latin, means "to teach." And it's through discipline that your child learns rules and limits. The structure provided helps her develop self-control, accountability, and positive self-esteem, and it also shows her how to accomplish these in spite of having a mood disorder. Some examples of discipline include letting natural consequences unfold, using rewards or incentives, and imposing penalties or time-outs for behaviors.

Punishment, on the other hand, is a negative response for an undesired behavior. Examples include yelling, hitting, lecturing, or shameful humiliation. Punishment focuses on what's been done *wrong* instead of what's been done *right*—and places the responsibility for behavioral management on the parent instead of encouraging the child to be responsible. Studies show that punishment leaves children with a poor self-image and a reduced sense of control over their lives.[6]

As with any chronic illness, a parent of a depressed child needs to take into consideration the child's depression, any special needs she has, and balance that while disciplining. Let's take a look at some tried and true ways to effectively discipline a depressed child.

- *See the behavior, not the disorder.* The best way to discipline your depressed child is to treat her need for structure, limits, and rules *just as you would any other child.* Despite her sadness or irritability, your child needs to learn responsibility, problem solving, and keeping commitments.
- *Break down tasks into smaller steps.* Because depression slows down thinking and action, help your child be successful with chores by breaking them down into smaller, more doable steps. If your preschooler has to clean up his "toys," tell him to start picking up the "cars" first. Then the "blocks." Now the "crayons." This sequential way of performing tasks helps him keep focus, promotes compliance, and, most of all, promotes self-esteem.
- *Adjust your time frame.* Along a similar line, build in some wiggle room for your child to get chores done. If you think it should take an hour for your teenager to clean her room, give her two. Make sure your expectations are balanced alongside the medical aspects of your child's depression.
- *Explain rules clearly.* By talking simply and clearly about how things run in the house, everyone in the family stays on the same page. Essentially,

your family will understand three things: 1) there will be rules everyone abides by in the home, 2) rewards and incentives will be used to help increase positive behaviors, and 3) consequences will be put in place for negative behaviors. This heads-up way of disciplining also helps your depressed child avoid using "the illness" to minimize expectations or manipulate you into letting things slide.

- *Be consistent.* Effective discipline requires a parent to be three things: Consistent. Consistent. Consistent. Parenting that is predictable gives ALL children a framework from which they find comfort. When families have routines—and parents mind its structure—children learn healthy skills.

- *Show unconditional love and support.* Though you might feel frustrated and overwhelmed at times, try to understand your child's thoughts and feelings—and support him without judgment. Remember that pediatric depression is a neurobiological illness that requires extra attention and intervention. Also, give yourself permission to be angry at the depression, but keep loving your child in spite of it.

CO-PARENTING ISSUES

Co-parenting, sometimes called *joint parenting* or *shared parenting*, is the experience of raising children as a single parent when separation or divorce occurs. Often a difficult process, co-parenting is greatly influenced by the reciprocal interactions of each parent.

If you are co-parenting a child with depression, you and your ex need to have empathy, patience, and open communication. This, of course, may not be an easy thing to achieve for couples who have encountered turbulent marital issues. Sometimes placing your child's needs over the marital disappointments may help coparenting be more successful. Consider using the following tips as a springboard to talk with your ex about better management of your depressed child.

- *Commit to making co-parenting an open dialogue with your ex.* Arrange to do this through email, texting, voicemail, letters, or face-to-face conversation. Studies show that there are many ways to collaboratively create structure for your depressed child, and that doing so increases her attainment of well-being.[7]

- *Discipline should be consistent and agreed upon at both households.* As much as he may fight it, a depressed child needs routine and structure. Issues such as mealtime, bedtime, and completing chores need to be consistent. The same goes for schoolwork and projects. As mentioned above, running a tight ship with discipline and structure creates a sense of security and predictability for him. When both households abide by this arrangement, your child knows that rules will be enforced no matter where he is. *"Just like at Mom's house, before we can go to the movies, you gotta get that bed made."*

- *Commit to positive talk around the house.* Make it a rule to try to talk positively about your ex. Angry and negative statements will reinforce your depressed child's sense of hopelessness and helplessness. Furthermore, if she sees you engaging in negative behaviors, she's unlikely to shift her own negative thinking patterns.

- *Create an extended family plan.* Negotiate and agree on the role extended family members will play if you or your ex cannot get your child to or from therapy. Same goes with medication—agree on who can dispense the doses. Arranging this ahead of time will offer consistency and predictability—two important elements in your depressed child's recovery.

- *Don't give in to guilt.* Divorce or separation are painful experiences and conjure up many kinds of emotions. Not being in your child's life on a full-time basis can cause you to convert your guilt into overindulgence. Understand how this plays out in unhealthy ways—and how granting wishes without limits is never good. Research shows that overindulgence can make your child become self-centered and have an unrealistic sense of entitlement.[8] As a parent, become attuned to the difference between what your depressed child *needs* versus *wants*, and help your ex understand this as well.

- *Seek supportive psychotherapy if necessary.* If you've tried and haven't found success getting your ex to work on these techniques, know that you don't have to go it alone. Consider involving yourself in psychotherapy to address how you can best parent your depressed child in spite of an uncooperative ex.

MAKE ROOM FOR YOU TIME

There's no doubt that being a parent is a full-time job. But caring for a child who has a depressive disorder adds even more demands to your role. Parenting is often fraught with stress, worry, and constant changes—and then there's the concern about how your child will fare in the future with this illness. The difficulties that come with parenting a child with depression have been given the term *caregiver strain*.[9]

Caring for your child will press heavily on your life not only as a parent but also as a person. This is why you need to find ways to soothe your own mind, body, and soul. If not, you run the risk of weakening your immune system, raising stress levels, and burning out.[10] And no one benefits from that. If you preach certain life rules to your depressed child, you'd better practice them too. Otherwise, a young child will get confused by your mixed messages. Or you might be on the receiving end of a finger-wagging, smirk-faced adolescent saying, "Do as I say, not as I do, huh?" An example, I'm sure, you don't want to set.

So, put your me-time hat on, read these suggestions, and be determined to make them happen.

- *Take off your superhero cape.* First things first. Realize that you can't *nor* should you be doing everything. The Superhero Mom or Dad mind-set is unachievable. If you are trying to do it all, you must retire the cape and shelve the utility belt. Be realistic about how much time and attention you can give to people and things in your life. Be mindful that not doing so can lead to burnout.
- *Delegate, then decompress.* Sometimes you need to figure out if you're truly the only one who can take of an issue regarding the care of your depressed child. This may mean delegating or relinquishing control. Can teachers help keep your child stay on course at school? Is your child ready to monitor his own medication needs? Can involving your child in a community sport or after-school hobby offer more than you

planning activities for him? Delegating gives you more time to rest, relax, and refuel.

- *Carving out couple time.* Many parents who care for a child with special needs get lost in daily routines. Parenting a child with depression also requires you put your spouse second as you tend to your child's needs first. Some partners manage their couple time well, but most partners feel lost or lonely, maybe even ignored—or just accept the situation as is. Research shows that scheduling time for date nights and sex recharges your love connection and leads to greater happiness in your coupledom.[11] Getting cozy also shows your children how to prioritize the importance of love and attachment. Remember, when you and your partner are happy and connected—in good and bad times—your children will feel happy and connected, too.

- *Plan scheduled breaks from parenting.* Don't forget to build time away from your parenting responsibilities. Get a babysitter, ask your partner to mind matters at home, or play hooky from work so you can connect with friends, take a class, pamper yourself, or just grab some alone time with a cup of coffee. Make having fun a chief goal so you can hold on to a sense of hope and optimism.

- *Confide in others.* Talking to others about what you're going through is a great way to let off steam. Be it a trusted friend, a loving family member, a parent support group, or a professional therapist, troubles shared are troubles halved.

- *Be proud of yourself.* Celebrate the fact that you're doing all you can to care for your depressed child. Whether you're a single parent or half of a parenting couple, be proud of the knowledge you've gained about mood disorders, the efforts you make to get all your child needs, and the sacrifices that sometimes occur along the way. Make sure to pat yourself on the back every now and again. You deserve it.

The following case study takes an indirect look at depression in children. It involved the treatment of a parent who needed guidance, encouragement, and tips for self-care. Once learned and used, they became the keys that unlocked a brittle and toxic family environment.

CASE STUDY: WAYNE

Wayne entered my office in a sharp suit and well-tailored overcoat. Referred by his physician, who was concerned about his stress level and high blood pressure, he readily took a seat, seemingly overwhelmed from his daily routine. Wayne was a high-power executive, who often traveled for work. Slightly grayed and weathered with wrinkles, he looked much older than his forty-two years. He was warm, smart, and verbal, and he appeared to have an easy way about him. The oldest of three children, he reported always being the caretaker of his family—a role he stepped into at age sixteen, after his father suddenly died. Despite the grief of his dad's death, he managed to graduate from high school and stayed home to go to college, so he could "look after his family." He found great success in college and graduate school, and he was recruited by a large business firm, where he slowly moved up the ladder—the same company where he remains to this day.

Divorced for three years, Wayne remained in the same town as his two sons, Matthew and Michael, and he made sure he never traveled on the scheduled weekends he had them. He described his divorce as "brutal" and that he was still involved in family court to enforce child visitation—something his ex-wife frequently sabotaged. His sons were assigned legal law guardians to help manage the family system, but the entire separation, divorce, and custody experience left Wayne feeling extremely depressed. And it appeared that his boys were struggling too, as both were in individual psychotherapy with separate therapists.

Wayne reported loving his sons deeply, and it upset him terribly to leave the marriage. He seemed as if he was a devoted father, arranging his schedule for not only visitations but also school plays, concerts, and teacher conferences. When we met, he was deliberating a job change, one that would have significantly less traveling, so when the boys were older he'd be able "to catch their high school sports."

After obtaining signed releases, I made the rounds touching base with his sons' therapists and law guardians. I came to learn that Wayne's son Michael was quite angry and defiant, while Matthew was significantly depressed. Wayne reported that parenting them was "difficult" despite the fact that he kept a firm but nurturing run of the house. Wayne reported not having a busy personal life, instead focusing just on "work and the boys" and not really having "time for that." Though he longed for time away from work and the kids, he hadn't taken a true vacation in four years.

Treatment objectives looked to address three areas of Wayne's life: home, work, and self. At home, we discovered that although he had good discipline techniques in place when it came to doing chores and finishing schoolwork, he was lax in some areas. He frequently spoke negatively about his ex in front of the boys and showed his exasperation about court proceedings. Sometimes he put the boys in the bind of choosing sides (a big no-no, he later learned). Though he kept the house clean and tidy, working so much left little time for him to shop for nutritious foods and snacks. As a result, the boys ate fast food or quick microwave dishes for virtually every meal when they were with him. It was clear that a lot of things could be managed better in these areas, with particular attention being paid to Wayne making time to tend to himself. I encouraged Wayne to realize that he wasn't really at his best with the kids—and probably not at his best at work—because he spent so little time resting and refueling.

"There's a reason they tell parents to put the oxygen mask on themselves first when air pressure changes on an airplane," I said to him. "You know why?"

Wayne nodded. "So you don't pass out before you help the kids."

The analogy kick-started a set of healthy changes in the following months of treatment. Wayne decided to shift jobs, giving him more time in town to tend to these newfound ideals. He told me that his local supermarket delivered food, so he was better at having healthy snacks and meals to cook when the boys were around. He tried to communicate openly with his ex via email, hoping to get her to work with the recommended structure, but he kept his cool when it never transpired. He also worked hard to curtail his anger and disappointment when court frustrated him or when his ex disrupted the visitation schedule. And he joined a gym, working out his aggravation and stress several times a week.

These changes were slow to take hold, but they did become routine as time progressed. Wayne shared that the boys seemed happier with him, and even enjoyed cooking a meal during their self-declared "boys night in." Contact with the therapists supported Wayne's report. Michael's therapist indicated a marked reduction in his irritability and anger. Matthew's therapist shared how his depression, while still there, was less much intense.

As for Wayne, he began looking less haggard and worn out, and the last few blood pressure check-ins showed better numbers. Happy to see all of these changes, I still wanted Wayne to have more personal time, more social experiences, love, intimacy, and even sex.

"What, like dating?" he asked me one day.

"Sure, why not?"

"Nah. Not ready to go down that road yet," he said with a smile. "But there are some hotties at the gym I like flirting with."

I grinned, realizing Wayne was already on his way.

Twenty Depression Myths Every Parent Should Know

What are myths? Why do they hold such power over public opinion? And how do they get started in the first place?

Myths are fabricated stories that attempt to define the existence of things. Myths have been long used in history, and they are most notably linked to the ancient Greeks for explaining things like thunder, fire, dreams, or war. For them, such natural experiences and physical phenomena resulted from the supernatural powers of specific gods and goddesses. These tales, of course, were never based in science, but were instead rationalized stories that offered comfort to the masses.

Fast forward several thousand years, and you'll find that myths continue to have a strong hold on humanity. It doesn't matter that science reveals the truths about certain long-held beliefs, such as that the Twinkie has an infinite shelf life (it doesn't—and remains edible for twenty-five days); that you shouldn't crack your knuckles because it can cause arthritis (science says no to this, too); or that shaving causes hair to grow back thicker (hair shafts appear coarser from shaving but do not actually grow in denser or with more volume). Though the aforementioned examples of myths are lighthearted in nature, there are other kinds of myths that, given enough room, can embed themselves in the fabric of society, leading to discrimination. In particular, myths that are race-based, gender-based, and sexual orientation–based generalize people instead of acknowledging diversity and uniqueness. And when it comes to individuals with mental illness, myths lead to not only discrimination but also stigma.

Stigma is a mark of disgrace or reproach assigned by society that identifies a child or adult as an outcast. One would think that the greatest obstacle a person has with mental illness comes from aspects of the disorder itself—but you'd be wrong if you thought that. Research shows the greatest problem preventing depressed children and adults from feeling better is stigma—the shame that surrounds having a mental illness.[1]

Despite the fact that evidence-based research shows that mental illness is a real medical disorder, stigma is on the rise instead of on the decline.[2] Stigma was expected to abate with increased knowledge of mental illness, but just the opposite occurred. Stigma has intensified over the past forty years even though understanding of what causes depression or bipolar moods has improved. Research has shown that knowledge of mental illness appears, by itself, not enough to dispel stigma.[3] Though we live in a century that brims with scientific discoveries and technological advances, many who live with depression feel the sting of discrimination that results from misconceptions of their illness. As a result, many won't seek treatment for fear that they'll be viewed in a negative way. The World Health Organization agrees and says that of the four hundred million people worldwide who are affected by mental illness, only 20 percent reach out for help.[4] Furthermore, the shameful stigma that cuts across nations and cultures around the world makes mental illness the largest and most destructive threat to health and well-being.[5]

MAKING SENSE OF STIGMA

I get all fired up when I talk or write about the issue of stigma regarding mental illness. I have felt the smack of it personally when ignorant people say hurtful things, joke insensitively, or even spout misguided information about mental illness. In truth, I have no patience for it—and generally jump right in to offer an appropriate correction to a discriminatory remark. Sometimes, I've been known to launch into a rather high-brow, research-specific tongue lashing to make my point. As a professional, I see how stigma keeps many children and adults away from treatment; how it deepens feelings of shame, as if having an illness is "wrong" or "bad"; and how the need to hide mental illness from others complicates feelings of self-worth.

When it comes to children, stigma will touch their lives in different ways. At very young ages, children aren't fully aware of the social discrimination out there regarding mental illness. Though they will be exposed to social experiences, cartoons, films, television, and radio programs that stigmatize mental illness,[6] in general, toddlers and preschoolers enter treatment without great feelings of shame. Things change, however, as children grow older. Their exposure and awareness to inaccurate and stereotypical myths are exponentially heightened. Social rules about shame regarding mental illness can be found virtually everywhere—from the kinds of slurs kids use on the playground, such as "crazy," "wacko," or "psycho," to adults' descriptions of another person's conduct as "maniac" or "nutjob." Those who need medication take "happy pills" or "psycho drugs." Gossip buzzes with negativity about "schizos" or "lunatics" when a mass tragedy strikes. Through these experiences, children are trained to believe that mental illness is an undesirable trait, a failure in character, and something to be feared. By the time children reach their teenage years, they have been so overly saturated with portrayals of the mentally ill as violent and dangerous that they fear self-identification with a subgroup that has been deemed "undesirable." They also reject any experience that may make them vulnerable to ridicule or exclusion, such as acknowledgment of their mood disorder, going for talk therapy, or considering medication.[7] Children often move through a process whereby they blame themselves for having depression, feel shame about that fact, and try to secrete away their illness, which leaves them feeling isolated—or, if the illness is known by others, it leaves them socially excluded. Simply said, the myths that persist teach children that it's very, very bad to have an association with mental illness.

Stigma doesn't only affect the life of your child. It can seep into the core of your soul, too. As a parent, you have the potential for finding yourself

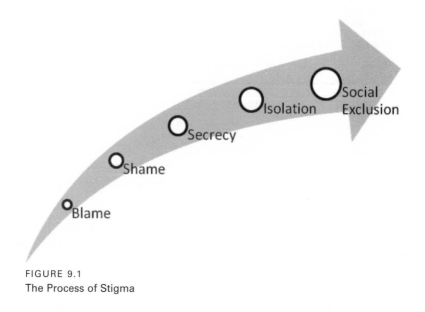

FIGURE 9.1
The Process of Stigma

socially disqualified from others because your child has a mood disorder. This is called *courtesy stigma* or *associative stigma*.[8] This kind of distorted thinking from uneducated others occurs because you share a genetic and environmental affiliation with a child who has mental illness. Because your son has depression or your daughter struggles with bipolar disorder, *you may have a disorder, too.* Along another line, ignorant people may believe you have a direct responsibility for your child having mental illness itself because you're a bad parent or have questionable genetic tendencies. Siblings can also experience this *stigma by association,* which devalues their status in social groups because their brother or sister has a mental illness. Like a contagious virus, others keep their distance from you, your child, and your child's siblings.

The psychology of understanding stigma can help you and your family cope with this social phenomenon.[9] Myths exist to defend against feelings of anxiety about things that elude or confuse people. Sometimes others use stigma as a way to offset feelings of their own insecurity—devaluing others to raise their own sense of worth. Some use stigma as a way to maintain self-preservation—carving out others who are perceived as threats.[10] Then there are people who have an unfiltered sense of reality, where their ignorance trumps reasonable facts. Whatever the reason, try to see stigma as "the other person's problem" and not a reality that you or your child have to live within.

One way to do this is to learn the myths about mental illness and become well versed in the facts that kick stigma to the curb. Not only does equipping yourself with these truths help you understand what depression truly is, it also builds confidence in yourself and your parenting—and ultimately creates greater self-esteem and self-worth in your child. When you think of stigma, think of the following:

> Watch your thoughts, for they become words.
> Watch your words, for they become actions.
> Watch your actions, for they become habits.
> Watch your habits, for they become character.
> Watch your character, for it becomes your destiny.
>
> —*Author Unknown*

This quote holds great insight for you, as a parent, and for your child. *The way you think becomes the world you live in.* When stigma hits with a barrel-chested bluster, just breathe deeply, find your center, rely on truths, and remember that there's no shame in living with mental illness.

DEPRESSION MYTHS

1. *Myth: Depression isn't a real medical problem.*

False: Depression is a very real illness that affects the emotional, social, behavioral, and physical health of children and adults. There are genetic and biological factors that predispose a child for depression, but life experiences also influence its development.

2. *Myth: Depression is not a common illness.*

False: Depression is more common than AIDS, cancer, and diabetes combined.

3. *Myth: Depression is only a problem of the Western industrialized world and not of developing countries.*

False: Depression affects children and adults in all cultures across the world. In fact, by the year 2020, depression will be the second leading cause of disability worldwide.

4. *Myth: Depression will go away on its own.*

False: A serious mental illness cannot be willed away or brushed aside with a change in attitude. Ignoring the problem doesn't give it the slip either. Depression is a serious, but treatable, illness, with a success rate of up to 80 percent for those who seek intervention.

5. *Myth: Nowadays, stigma for children and teens living with depression has declined.*

False: Though evidence-based research has shown depression is a real illness, stigma is on the rise instead of on the decline. There is so much shame regarding mental illness that statistics show only one in five actually seek treatment. Studies have shown that knowledge of depression appears insufficient to dispel stigma. What does reduce stigma? Learning about positive and inspiring stories of people living successfully with depression.

6. *Myth: Pediatric depression is not a major health concern.*

False: Pediatric depression is a significant health concern. In the United States, evidence suggests that 4 percent of preschool-aged children, 5 percent of school-aged children, and 11 percent of adolescents meet the criteria for major depression.

7. *Myth: Good parents can always detect if their child is depressed.*

False: Most children who suffer with depression keep their thoughts and feelings masked. The only way for parents to understand depression is to be aware of age-specific behaviors and symptoms. Depression is not a result of bad parenting.

8. *Myth: A depressed child is a loner.*

False: As previously mentioned, children often mask their depression. So a child can present as happy, social, or untroubled on the outside, though internally she is struggling terribly with negative thoughts and despairing feelings.

9. *Myth: Children with mental illness are prone to violence.*

False: Research shows that children with mental illness are more likely to be the victim of violence than be the cause of it.

10. *Myth: Antidepressants are "addictive."*

False: Antidepressants are not addictive. A child will not "crave" an antidepressant.

11. *Myth: Antidepressants are a "quick fix" and don't really cure depression.*

False: One thing antidepressants surely aren't is quick. Most take a minimum of four to six weeks to work. Antidepressant medications adjust brain chemistry, which will improve mood and cognition and allow for healthier lifestyle choices and problem solving.

12. *Myth: Antidepressants will change your child's personality.*

False: Antidepressants normalize the ranges of moods in children who have a mood disorder—and will not change your child's personality.

13. *Myth: Once your child starts taking antidepressants, he will be on them for the rest of his life.*

False: The majority of children who take antidepressant medication will stop their prescription in a careful and modified manner when recovery from depression occurs. This clinical state of recovery takes about a year or so to achieve.

14. *Myth: Talking about depression gives kids ideas and makes things worse.*

False: Talking about depression with your child actually helps to reduce symptoms. Support and encouragement through open communication are significantly meaningful. This lets your child know he's not alone and is loved and cared for.

15. *Myth: Telling on a child who is depressed and suicidal is betraying a trust. If she truly wants help, she will ask for it or get it somehow.*

    False: Depression depletes energy and self-esteem. As a result, depression often interferes with a child's ability to reach out to others. While your child may be angry if a friend tells about her depression, or if you seek professional counsel as to what to do, her feelings will be of short duration. Most children are relieved that others intervened on their behalf once the grip of depression eases.

16. *Myth: The risk of suicide for children is greatly exaggerated.*

    False: Suicide is the third leading cause of death in adolescents ages fifteen to twenty-four, and it is the sixth leading cause of death in children ages five to fourteen. Suicide is significantly linked to depression, so early diagnosis and treatment of pediatric depression are extremely important.

17. *Myth: Children and teens don't use suicide hotlines—and neither do parents.*

    False: Suicide hotlines are being used now more than ever. In fact, over $55 million of federal grant money has been used to expand hotline training and programs. Parents call for information and resources and children and teens reach out to help a friend or to stop themselves from self-destructive thoughts. Even veterans, active and retired, are calling hotlines such as 800-273-TALK, 800-SUICIDE, and 877-YOUTHLINE.

18. *Myth: My pediatrician says my child's moodiness is just a phase—and not to worry.*

    False: General practitioners and pediatricians, while trained in aspects of mental illness, are not specialists. If you're on the receiving end of a *don't-worry-it's-just-a-stage* response from your family physician, seek a second opinion from a mental health specialist.

19. *Myth: When a depressed child refuses help, there's nothing parents can do.*

False: If your child refuses to go to talk therapy or take medication, there are things you can do. You can seek therapy with a trained mental health specialist to learn how to help your child in spite of the fact that he won't attend sessions. In a crisis situation, you can drive your child to the nearest hospital emergency room, or contact family, friends, or the local police for assistance in getting him there.

20. *Myth: Seriously depressed people cannot lead productive lives.* ·

False: Many with depression can live full, productive lives. In fact, many high-profile people, including president Abraham Lincoln, writer J. K. Rowling, artist Michelangelo, actor Harrison Ford, choreographer Alvin Ailey, actress Courteney Cox, entrepreneur Richard Branson, prime minister Winston Churchill, rocker Bruce Springsteen, and baseball player Ken Griffey Jr., have been very successful in their chosen professions.

A HEALTHY PERSPECTIVE

It has been said that living with a mental illness is all about perspective.[11] What's important for you as a parent of a depressed child is to ground yourself in the reality of science, not myth, and to trust your instincts when it comes to what's best for your child because no one knows her strengths and weaknesses better than you. With your help, you can empower your child and increase his comfort in managing his depression. Fostering this healthy perspective inoculates him with self-confidence, teaches him that illness doesn't define a person, and allows him to seek treatment later on in life if it's needed.

Dealing with the realities of living with depression can take some time for children to understand. It isn't easy adjusting patterns of thinking, learning how to regulate emotions, shifting negative habits into more positive ones, taking medication consistently, and dealing with the stigma that bears down from time to time. In the case study that follows, you'll see how a depressed patient learned to fortify herself with truths and facts so that her family's stigmatizing ways couldn't keep her down.

CASE STUDY: LINDA

Linda doesn't remember much of her childhood. What she does recall paints a picture of an extremely depressed child who grew up feeling invisible. One of ten children, Linda appeared to float in and around family members, never really feeling connected to them. Her memories were filled with feeling states that were hard to endure. Linda recalled how great sadness, insecurity, and anxiety filled her life. Though she strived to always be a good girl, following rules, trying to do well in school, and excelling in music, she was often overlooked or unrecognized among family members. As a result, Linda felt guilt about things she thought or did and self-blame followed her like a shadow. She frequently shared that the loneliest feeling in the world for her was being in a room full of people and feeling like she wasn't there.

Linda's father was a well-educated man, and her mother was a secretary. Though Linda never went without material things in her large family, it appeared that she greatly missed a tremendous amount of emotional nurturance from her parents and siblings. One of the reasons for this void was the death of an older sister from an illness. Though Linda was a small girl when this happened, the traumatic event arrested the family dynamics. As is often the case, parts of her parents and siblings died along with her sister. A lot of the early work Linda and I did in treatment focused on helping her make sense of why her parents were so detached and how that factored into her helpless feelings, her hopeless thoughts, and her overwhelming feelings of guilt. Gaining insight from her family history, we learned that every member of her family lived in denial about many things, from the death of her sister to sexual abuse and severe drug and alcohol addictions that plagued certain family members. The code for the family was that no one talked about these things. And if someone brought it up, it was "knocked down" right away.

When Linda found it increasingly difficult to manage her depression and suicidal thinking took hold, she needed to be hospitalized. It was during her first hospitalization that she encountered the stigma of mental illness from family members. Up until then, she was able to mask her sadness and tuck away the thoughts that tormented her. But now, her crisis couldn't remain unseen. One family member after the other conveyed the message that she was of *weak character, lazy,* or *just not trying hard enough.* Some of her siblings questioned the kind of treatments she was undergoing—planting ideas that taking medicine was *addictive,* that therapy was a *crutch,* and so many more myths. At first, it was hard to convince Linda that her family was wrong, because for the first time in her life, she was being seen, and she wanted their concern to have meaning, for it to hold value. But Linda soon realized that their hurtful words and controlling ways weren't helpful at all. In fact, they made her feel worse.

Linda and I worked on helping her understand the power stigma has on her recovery. Whereas before she understood how genetics and life experiences shaped her depression, the myths she was hearing got her wondering if her illness *was truly real at all.*

"Maybe I'm just being too sensitive?" she'd say.

With a lot of work and effort on her part, Linda became more empowered and confident, knowing what the truths were when it came to her depression. Not only did she work in sessions on learning facts and figures, she also read a lot online and became well versed in medication and psychotherapy. Linda grew braver when she was with her large family, taking on brothers or sisters who said stupid things or tried to make her feel bad. She educated her parents about mental illness, too, and though denial and minimization occurred, Linda knew she wasn't invisible anymore.

Some years later, Linda required another hospitalization. This time, she limited who could visit, was prepared to deal with inappropriate comments, and became more assertive in what she needed and wanted from family members. The manner in which she handled her recovery was inspiring to witness. I knew it wasn't easy for her to combat the persistent nature of her family's dynamics. I also knew how very much she needed their love and acceptance, and how she and I needed to be realistic about that in our treatment goals. What seemed to keep Linda tuned and channeled to her health were the numbers, statistics, research, and science that explained mental illness. Like anchors, they grounded her during the turbulent refusals that came when her family tried to refute the reality of her illness.

As a parent with her own children, Linda has created an open forum where each child is not only seen but also celebrated. She struggles with significant depression sometimes, but uses her skills and her medications to help her get through episodes. Armed with scientific data and personal life experience, she is now a go-to expert for her very large, extended family. By educating others, addressing stigma, dispelling ignorance, and highlighting what is being denied, she not only validates that she's smart and knowledgeable but also declares that she doesn't have to hide in shame because she has depression.

Linda has so much to offer that she has given thought to becoming a trained member of the local suicide hotline. She has also considered going back to school to get a degree in psychology. Every time she mentions these dreams to me, I smile and tell her she'd be great. I know that she has what it takes to do all these things.

And that she'll be seen, valued, and loved.

10

Planning for the Future

Learning that your child has unipolar or bipolar disorder is an intensely emotional experience. Many parents and caregivers who recognize their child needs immediate or ongoing intervention can be overwhelmed in a tidal wave of feelings—including fear, confusion, and worry. Studies show that a parent's experience of a child's mental illness can include an intense and persistent sadness—a term called *chronic sorrow*.[1] And then there are feelings of loss. Not just the immediate loss felt in the face of your child's diagnosis, but also something more. A loss that is complex and ongoing, not like the kind of loss experienced by bereavement—but the kind of loss that has no predictable end.[2]

SETTING REALISTIC GOALS

There is no doubt that tremendous psychological strain is felt by families who have a child with mental illness. What makes this even more heart wrenching is the cyclical nature of unipolar and bipolar disorders, the "sometimes" experience of your child having good moments—with periods of her former self glimmering wonderfully in front of you—only for the illness to surge again and take that away.

When thinking of your child's future, it's important to remember the trajectory of his illness. It's vital to note the intensity of the disorder. Mild and moderate cases of *any illness* often move better through life than serious or profound ones. Understand the chronicity as well as the cyclical patterns of your child's depression. Has your child's depression reached a response level at which symptoms have reduced? Has he advanced to the clinical level at which recovery has occurred? Has a full remission been experienced? What about recurrence—has he had another onset? Is there a treatment-resistance depression operating? Adherence to treatment is also extremely imperative. While as a young child you may have been able to direct his compliance regarding going to therapy or taking medication, as he gets older, perhaps you can't. Once you paint a picture of your child's unique experience with depression, you can work toward creating healthy expectations. Grounding yourself in this way will help design more realistic hope about your child's future.

The future for a child with mild or moderate depression is that he or she needs to be aware of symptoms and how to interrupt the onset from deepening further. Most adults who were children with depression work on their skills or, if necessary, go back into treatment to bolster them. Sometimes a return to medication occurs, sometimes not. They may have stress-related issues at home or work and encounter social and relational difficulties. There may be physical and somatic concerns presenting as well. Overall, these issues do not exceedingly impair their ability to meet life's challenges.

Adults who were children with severe or profound unipolar or bipolar depression face greater odds in life. According to research, approximately 3 percent of American adults fall into this description of severe mental illness.[3] Whether the severity of the disorder comes from a treatment-resistant depression or noncompliance in following treatment recommendations, adults with unipolar or bipolar depression are at risk for social, cognitive, and behavioral deficits that may lead to inadequate health and self-care practices.[4] Having a meaningful work, social, or personal life without challenge is not a likely outcome. This will cause such anguish for parents. The unimaginable thought of *who will look after my child once I'm gone* begins to grow. Like a bone in the throat, the thought chokes your confidence and floods you with worry.

There are many ways for an adult with significant depression to find support, guidance, and caretaking. Services such as group homes, co-ops, and independent housing that stress independent living can help. In the United States, many are provided by government assistance or are covered by long-term care insurance, health insurance, or funds placed in trust. In Canada, the United Kingdom, Ireland, Australia, and New Zealand, the local housing authority or council housing offices will assist in finding programs and housing.[5] Local, national, and international mental health associations offer enormous support in this regard—and will help you to never feel alone in this journey.

AVAILABLE CARE OPTIONS

If your child moves from adolescence into adulthood with severe or profound symptoms, there are a number of care options you can consider. Remember to find what suits your child's needs best—and what works best with your needs as well. Dr. Deborah Elbaum,[6] a contributing writer for Care.com, offers the following suggestions:

- *Family members.* Many adult children live at home with family members as their primary care providers.
- *Home health aides or personal care attendants.* Depending on the child's level of need, these providers come into the home to help family members in a variety of ways.
- *Community-based homes and supported living arrangements.* Adults living in group homes enjoy some independence but receive support as necessary depending on their needs.
- *Independent living arrangements.* Depending on their situation, some adults may be able to live independently with some form of additional support. For example, they may need someone to help them for a few hours a day with activities of daily living, transportation, meals, and other things.
- *Day programs.* Once they are no longer attending school, adults can benefit from day programs appropriate for their level of ability. Providing

structure to the day through a variety of educational services, these programs help adults work on life skills while offering social opportunities.

- *Long-term care facilities.* Some adult children with special needs require extensive support around the clock. In cases such as this, parents may feel their child's needs are best served in a long-term, live-in care facility.
- *Assistive technology.* There's a wealth of assistive technology, from software to sports gear, which may help your adult child be more independent.

THE IMPORTANCE OF HOPE

The definition of *hope* is an inspiration, an aim. When your child was first born, you had many hopes for her. As she grew older, you may have needed to shift or redefine them. And once learning that she had a depressive disorder, maybe you needed to redesign them all over again. Just as you moved through the stages of grief when you first learned of your child's diagnosis, the same step-by-step grieving will happen when you think about her future. The important thing is to hold tight to the love you have for your child as you come to accept a different set of hopes. Studies cite the crucial importance of parents who ground themselves in realistic hope as being the single most influential factor in bringing meaning to their child's life.[7]

As a parent, your journey with your child as he grows will be filled with many challenges. With realistic expectations, the goal is for you to also have moments of joy and happiness, too. Let's take a look at some tips to help you manage this difficult, yet important, journey:

1. *Remember to see your child, not the disorder.* As mentioned before, how you perceive your child and how you define her depression will greatly impact your relationship with her. Strive to see your child as a whole person, not just her illness.
2. *Realize that your child's needs will change over time.* As your child ages, so, too, will the quality and quantity of his needs. This will require you to be flexible not only when it comes *to coordinating care, but also in adjusting your own emotional expectations.*

3. *Know when to step in and when to let go.* Being a parent of a child with unipolar or bipolar disorder will test your tendency to overprotect. Try your best to choose when you'll intervene to help your child as she works through problems in school, work, home, or with others. Stepping in too much will create dependency and prevent her from finding out what her optimal skill set is, and staying on the sidelines too much may constrict her confidence. Striking that right balance will take some time, and once you find it, expect that it may tug at your heartstrings nonetheless.

4. *Consider setting up long-term care.* Whether it's calling on government-funded disability services or private long-term care insurance policies, realize that not doing so can create unnecessary chaos when you're no longer able to care for your child. This is, without question, one of the most difficult decisions a parent can ever make. Reach out to family, friends, or more formal support from national mental health organizations, legal and financial advisors, or therapists so you're not alone during this process.

5. *Your child should be empowered to have his own life, and so should you.* This is something all parents face when their children set out in adulthood. What makes this particular experience harder for you is that your adult child may make choices that aren't healthy or productive. When this happens, try to honor your child's decision and work within its limitations. If your child works to reach his optimal potential, encourage him to continue making a meaningful life for himself. And remember that you, too, deserve to have a life that empowers you, feeds you, and brings you purpose.

I thought I would share myself as a case study for this chapter's example. Much of my early life with depression was met with reluctance and resistance from my parents. It was hard for me to understand their reactions, but with age and experience I realized what was going on. And with the insight you've now gained from this chapter, so will you.

CASE STUDY: DEBORAH

"You're still going to therapy?" my mother asks, her hands on her hips.

"Of course," I say, with a roll of my eyes.

My mother was fifty-two—the age I am now as I write this—when that moment occurred. I was almost twenty-three, and still working with the therapist who saved me from a suicidal despair. I can see myself sitting at the round oak table my father built in the kitchen, a cup of tea in hand. My mother's words pierce like a hot spray of buckshot, but I try not to let her know I'm hurt. Instead, I look at her with a side-eyed, incredulous glance. I think to myself that either she's suddenly in denial over my suicide attempt a few years back or in her mind she believes the crisis is over.

"Well, I'm getting tired of paying for these sessions," she said, writing out the check in hard, swift strokes.

When I was in recovery from my major depression, I never really considered how it truly touched my parents' world. I was busy working at my treatment and trying to meet the challenges of college, work, and my social life. It wasn't easy, but I was getting there.

It always upset me when my mother said things like that, as if she was intolerant of my needs or ashamed of them. I vowed after college was done, I'd take over payments for my therapy sessions.

And as soon as I landed a full-time job as a school psychologist, I did.

But there still were times when she'd make a comment about me needing therapy.

As time went on, I moved out of my home, fell in love, and got married—all while continuing in talk therapy. I accepted that I needed weekly sessions to prevent severe depressions from returning. I was fine with that, even if my parents bristled at that fact. In the ten years that came to pass since my suicide attempt, I learned valuable skills in therapy. And when time arrived to end treatment, I felt strong, ready, and glad. I remember my parents being very happy when I told them.

"Well, you worked real hard," my dad said. "It shows."

My mother said nothing and just smiled.

In the years that passed, I made decisions that took my career path away from working for others (school settings) to working for myself (private practice). It was clearly different from the seven-hour-day, nine-months-with-summers-off job I had as a school psychologist. Though I was working more days and seemingly more hours, I loved being my own boss. I felt such freedom in setting my work hours in spurts throughout the day—two patients here, two patients there, teaching a class, lunch out with some errands if needed, followed by some time for writing or another two patients here and two patients there. Not working a solid seven hours in a steady "work mode" suited my emotional and physical needs. I had a passion for my work and felt fulfilled in every aspect of it.

My parents, however, didn't like my move from the structure of the school setting. They "worried" I was setting myself up for a crash. Working more didn't make sense to them. *Haven't you learned that you need to balance your life, to keep things simple, so another depressive episode doesn't happen? Why are you doing so many things? Why would you give up a job that was paying for your health care insurance?* They also grumbled loudly—and often—that leaving the school district also ended the benefit of a cushy pension. They called me foolish. Short-sighted. And sometimes if the subject came up and I rubbed them the wrong way with my *it's-my-life-leave-me-alone* answer, they'd call me stupid.

It didn't matter that I was making a good living, that I was saving money, or had self-employed retirement accounts set up and good health insurance through my husband's job. It frustrated me that they continued to be so critical of how I was conducting my life. I felt so alone and misunderstood. So I began sharing less and less with them.

Some years later, I crashed. Again. I fell into another double depression, this time shortly after my daughter was born. It didn't take me by surprise, as I was mindful of it, knowing that a previous major depressive episode heightened the likelihood of a postpartum onset. As I began treatment again, I added medication. It was a relatively new way of treating depression back in the 1990s—and I was open to including it in my treatment plan.

"Why you taking those?" my dad asked, upset.

"Because I think they'll really help," I said.

My mother had a pained look on her face and hissed one of her long, drawn-out sighs. I imagined she was thinking *here we go again.*

It didn't take long for feelings of shame to hit me. A sudden realization, in the space between two breaths, that I was disappointing them once again.

It would be a long time before I realized they were experiencing something very, very different from what I was imagining. Becoming a parent myself helped me reflect on my parents' brusque reactions. I realized that behind their clipped remarks was great sadness. There was also great worry and concern for my future. They wanted things to be as easy as possible for me because I struggled with depression. They wanted security for me—and for their own peace of mind. They never wanted to see me fragile, weak, or worn to the point of not wanting to live anymore ever again. Working nine months a year sounded less pressured to them than working year-round. Working a short day from 9 a.m. to 3 p.m. appeared less overwhelming than seeing a patient at 9 a.m. and ending my workday with a patient at 9 p.m., and a state pension could allow me to retire young and live well. And I'd also have guaranteed health insurance.

My parents lived with a chronic sense of grief—something I needed to honor and respect. It's not that they were ashamed of me. It's not that I failed them. The irritation and anger I saw were rooted in a sense of helplessness. They grieved the loss of me having an easier life, one that didn't require so many adjustments and accommodations.

Over the years, I've worked with my parents to help them see that I have a rich and meaningful life in spite of the fact that I live with depression. I tell them that the way I've configured my life fits better than the ideal they sometimes hold in their head of what might be best for me. I acknowledge their sorrows and worries, as they do with my needs and wishes. I share more, talk more, and show more to them— so they can truly know who I am in spite of my depression. It's true, I suffer through side effects from medication, need to modify my social and work life in ways that don't overwhelm me, and struggle from time to time. Through our more open communications, I know they don't worry like they used to. In fact, they reveal more candidly how proud they are of me and all of my achievements—great and small. Which, of course, feels wonderful.

But every now and again, I'll catch my mom with that pained look on her face. Whether she sees me while I'm taking a dose of my medication or teary-eyed about something that's overwhelming me, I don't get angry at her. Instead, I take her hand and squeeze it gently. Lovingly.

"I'm good, Ma," I say.

And I truly am.

Appendix A

Medication Side-Effect Checklist for Children and Adolescents

Child's Name: _____ Date: _____
Name of Medication: _____ Dosage: _____
☐ Before Medication Begins ☐ After Medication (__ weeks/months/years)

PHYSICAL SIDE EFFECTS

Please circle the level of each behavior you have observed in your child.

Bites nails	none	mild	moderate	severe
Dizziness	none	mild	moderate	severe
Drowsiness	none	mild	moderate	severe
Explosive outbursts	none	mild	moderate	severe
Fidgetiness	none	mild	moderate	severe
Forgetfulness	none	mild	moderate	severe
Gastrointestinal distress	none	mild	moderate	severe
Headaches	none	mild	moderate	severe
Nervousness	none	mild	moderate	severe
Nightmares	none	mild	moderate	severe
No appetite	none	mild	moderate	severe
Pacing/restless	none	mild	moderate	severe
Physically aggressive	none	mild	moderate	severe
Prone to crying	none	mild	moderate	severe
Self-destructive	none	mild	moderate	severe
Sleeping long hours	none	mild	moderate	severe
Stomachaches	none	mild	moderate	severe
Temper tantrums	none	mild	moderate	severe
Trouble sleeping	none	mild	moderate	severe
Verbally abusive	none	mild	moderate	severe
Violent	none	mild	moderate	severe

Child's Name: _____   Date: _____
Name of Medication: _____   Dosage: _____
☐ Before Medication Begins ☐ After Medication (__ weeks/months/years)

EMOTIONAL SIDE EFFECTS

Please circle the level of each behavior you have observed in your child.

Absence of emotions	none	mild	moderate	severe
Apathy	none	mild	moderate	severe
Behaving differently than usual	none	mild	moderate	severe
Disconnected from friends	none	mild	moderate	severe
Disconnected from school	none	mild	moderate	severe
Dulled emotions	none	mild	moderate	severe
Emotional detachment	none	mild	moderate	severe
Flattened speech	none	mild	moderate	severe
Ignoring responsibilities	none	mild	moderate	severe
Inability to cry	none	mild	moderate	severe
Loss of motivation	none	mild	moderate	severe
Loss of playfulness	none	mild	moderate	severe
Loss of self-care	none	mild	moderate	severe
Reduced intensity of happiness	none	mild	moderate	severe
Reports feeling different	none	mild	moderate	severe
Sudden shift in character	none	mild	moderate	severe
Thoughts of self-harm	none	mild	moderate	severe
Trouble feeling loved	none	mild	moderate	severe
Unhelpful	none	mild	moderate	severe

Appendix B

High-Profile People with Mood Disorders*

Name	Prominence	Diagnosis
John Quincy Adams	American President	Depression
Andre Agassi	American Tennis Player	Depression
Alvin Ailey	American Choreographer	Bipolar
Buzz Aldrin	American Astronaut	Depression
Claus Von Amsberg	Prince of Netherlands	Depression
Hans Christian Andersen	Danish Writer	Depression
Louie Anderson	American Comedian	Depression
Shawn Andrews	American Football Player	Depression
Ann-Margret	American Actor	Depression
Adam Ant	British Singer	Bipolar
Vin Baker	American Basketball Player	Depression
Alec Baldwin	American Actor	Depression
Brigitte Bardot	French Actor	Depression
James M. Barrie	Scottish Writer	Depression
Drew Barrymore	American Actor	Depression
Ludwig van Beethoven	German Composer	Bipolar
Ingmar Bergman	Swedish Film Director	Depression

*As previously published in Deborah Serani, *Living with Depression* (Lanham, MD: Rowman & Littlefield, 2011).

Name	Prominence	Diagnosis
Irving Berlin	American Composer	Depression
Hector Berlioz	French Composer	Bipolar
Maurice Bernard	American Actor	Bipolar
Leonard Bernstein	American Composer	Depression
Halle Berry	American Actor	Depression
Valerie Bertinelli	American Actor	Depression
William Blake	British Poet	Depression
David Bohm	British Physicist	Depression
Kjell Magne Bondevik	Prime Minister of Norway	Depression
Clara Bow	American Actor	Depression
Steven Bowditch	Australian Golfer	Depression
David Bowie	British Singer	Depression
Susan Boyle	British Singer	Depression
Lorraine Bracco	American Actor	Depression
Terry Bradshaw	American Football Player	Depression
Zach Braff	American Actor	Depression
Lord Melvyn Bragg	British Writer	Depression
Jo Brand	British Comedian	Bipolar
Russell Brand	British Comedian	Bipolar
Marlon Brando	American Actor	Depression
Sir Richard Branson	British Entrepreneur	Depression
Charlotte Brontë	British Author	Depression
Frank Bruno	British Boxer	Depression
Art Buchwald	American Writer	Bipolar
Delta Burke	American Actor	Depression
Carol Burnett	American Comedian	Depression
Robert Burton	British Academic	Depression
Tim Burton	British Director	Bipolar
Barbara Bush	American First Lady	Depression
Gabriel Byrne	Irish Actor	Depression
Lord Byron	British Poet	Depression
Beverley Callard	British Actor	Depression
Robert Campeau	Canadian Entrepreneur	Bipolar
Jose Canseco	American Baseball Player	Depression

Name	Prominence	Diagnosis
Drew Carey	American Comedian	Depression
Jim Carrey	American Actor	Depression
Dick Cavett	American Talk Show Host	Depression
Mary Chapin-Carpenter	American Country Singer	Depression
David Chase	American Writer	Depression
Lawton Chiles	American Governor	Depression
Agatha Christie	British Writer	Depression
Winston Churchill	British Prime Minister	Depression
Eric Clapton	British Musician	Depression
Dick Clark	American Entrepreneur	Depression
John Cleese	British Actor	Depression
Rosemary Clooney	American Singer	Bipolar
Jessie Close	Sister of actor Glenn Close	Depression
Leonard Cohen	Canadian Musician	Depression
Natalie Cole	American Singer	Depression
Judy Collins	American Singer	Depression
Pat Conroy	American Writer	Depression
Calvin Coolidge	American President	Depression
Francis Ford Coppola	American Film Director	Bipolar
Patricia Cornwell	American Writer	Bipolar
Noel Coward	British Writer/Composer	Bipolar
Simon Cowell	British Record Producer	Depression
Courtney Cox	American Actor	Postpartum
Michael Crichton	American Writer	Depression
Sheryl Crow	American Musician	Depression
Billy Crystal	American Comedian/Actor	Depression
John Daly	American Golfer	Bipolar
Rodney Dangerfield	American Comedian	Depression
Ray Davies	British Musician	Bipolar
Jack Dee	British Comedian	Depression
Edgar Degas	French Painter	Depression
Ellen DeGeneres	American Comedian	Depression
Sandy Denton	American Singer	Postpartum
John Denver	American Musician	Depression

Name	Prominence	Diagnosis
Charles Dickens	British Writer	Depression
Emily Dickinson	American Poet	Depression
Benjamin Disraeli	British Prime Minister	Depression
Scott Donie	American Olympic Diver	Depression
Gaetano Donizetti	Italian Composer	Bipolar
Fyodor Dostoevsky	Russian Writer	Depression
Mike Douglas	American TV Host	Depression
Theodore Dreiser	American Writer	Depression
Richard Dreyfuss	American Actor	Bipolar
Kitty Dukakis	First Lady of Massachusetts	Bipolar
Patty Duke	American Actor	Bipolar
Kirsten Dunst	American Actor	Depression
Adam Duritz	American Singer	Depression
Thomas Eagleton	American Senator	Depression
Thomas Eakins	American Painter	Depression
George Eliot	British Writer	Depression
T. S. Eliot	American Writer	Depression
James Ellroy	American Writer	Depression
Ralph Waldo Emerson	American Writer	Depression
James Farmer	American Civil Rights Leader	Depression
William Faulkner	American Writer	Depression
Jules Feiffer	American Cartoonist	Depression
Craig Ferguson	Scottish Comedian	Bipolar
Sarah Ferguson	British Duchess of York	Depression
Carrie Fisher	American Actor	Bipolar
Eddie Fisher	American Actor	Depression
F. Scott Fitzgerald	American Writer	Depression
Kevin Foley	South Australia Deputy Premier	Depression
Harrison Ford	American Actor	Depression
Tom Ford	American Fashion Designer	Depression
Stephen Foster	American Composer	Depression
Connie Francis	American Singer	Bipolar

Name	Prominence	Diagnosis
Stephen Fry	British Actor	Bipolar
Peter Gabriel	British Musician	Depression
John Kenneth Gailbraith	Canadian Economist	Depression
James Garner	American Actor	Depression
Paul Gascoigne	British Footballer	Bipolar
Paul Gauguin	French Painter	Depression
John Paul Getty	American Philanthropist	Depression
John Gibson	Irish Pianist	Bipolar
Mel Gibson	American Actor	Bipolar
Sir John Gielgud	British Actor	Depression
Kendall Gill	American Basketballer	Depression
Matthew Good	Canadian Musician	Bipolar
Tipper Gore	Wife of Vice President	Depression
Francisco de Goya	Spanish Painter	Depression
Amy Grant	American Singer	Postpartum
Cary Grant	American Actor	Depression
Graham Greene	British Writer	Bipolar
Tim Gunn	American Fashion Consultant	Depression
Dorothy Hamill	American Olympic Skater	Depression
Linda Hamilton	American Actor	Bipolar
Susie Favor Hamilton	American Olympic Runner	Depression
Tyler Hamilton	American Olympic Bicyclist	Depression
John Hamm	American Actor	Depression
George F. Handel	German Composer	Bipolar
Angie Harmon	American Actor	Postpartum
Pete Harnish	American Baseball Player	Depression
Mariette Hartley	American Actor	Bipolar
Juliana Hatfield	American Singer	Depression
Stephen Hawking	American Physicist	Depression
Paige Hemmis	American TV Host	Depression
Audrey Hepburn	American Actor	Depression
Hermann Hesse	Swiss Writer	Depression
Dame Kelly Holmes	British Olympic Runner	Depression

Name	Prominence	Diagnosis
Sir Anthony Hopkins	British Actor	Depression
Victor Hugo	French Writer	Depression
Hulk Hogan	American Wrestler	Depression
Henrik Ibsen	Norwegian Playwright	Depression
Natalie Imbruglia	Australian Singer/Actress	Depression
La India	Latin Salsa Singer	Depression
Jack Irons	American Musician	Bipolar
Janet Jackson	American Singer	Depression
Kay Redfield Jamison	American Psychologist	Bipolar
Thomas Jefferson	American President	Depression
Billy Joel	American Musician	Depression
Sir Elton John	British Singer	Bipolar
Andrew Johns	British Rugby Player	Bipolar
Daniel Johns	Australian Musician	Depression
Russ Johnson	American Baseball Player	Depression
Ashley Judd	American Actor	Depression
Franz Kafka	German Writer	Depression
Karen Kain	Canadian Ballerina	Depression
Kerry Katona	British Singer	Bipolar
Danny Kaye	American Actor	Depression
John Keats	British Poet	Depression
Patrick Kennedy	American Congressman	Bipolar
Ted Kennedy	American Senator	Depression
Jack Kerouac	American Writer	Depression
Alicia Keys	American Musician	Depression
Margot Kidder	American Actor	Bipolar
Søren Kierkegaard	Danish Philosopher	Depression
Gelsey Kirkland	American Ballerina	Depression
John Kirwan	New Zealand Rugby Player	Depression
Beyonce Knowles	American Singer	Depression
Joey Kramer	American Musician	Depression
Kris Kristopherson	American Musician	Depression
Julie Krone	American Jockey	Depression
Akira Kurosawa	Japanese Film Director	Depression

Name	Prominence	Diagnosis
Lady Gaga	American Musician	Depression
Pat LaFontaine	American Hockey Player	Depression
Hugh Laurie	British Actor	Depression
Peter Nolan Lawrence	British Writer	Bipolar
Frances Lear	American TV Producer	Bipolar
Vivien Leigh	British Actor	Bipolar
John Lennon	British Musician	Depression
Neil Lennon	British Footballer	Bipolar
Denise L'Estrange-Corbet	New Zealand Fashion Designer	Depression
David Letterman	American Comedian	Depression
Jennifer Lewis	American Actor	Bipolar
Meriwether Lewis	American Explorer	Depression
Abraham Lincoln	American President	Depression
Joshua Logan	American Playwright	Bipolar
Federico Garcia Lorca	Spanish Poet/Playwright	Depression
Robert Lowell	American Poet	Depression
Salvador Luria	Italian Nobel Laureate	Depression
Gustav Mahler	Austrian Composer	Depression
Norman Mailer	American Writer	Depression
Margaret Manning	American Psychologist	Depression
Henri Matisse	French Artist	Depression
Brian May	British Musician	Depression
Sir Paul McCartney	British Musician	Depression
Gary McDonald	Australian Actor	Depression
Sarah McLachlan	Canadian Musician	Depression
Kristy McNichol	American Actor	Bipolar
John Mellencamp	American Musician	Depression
Herman Melville	American Writer	Depression
Burgess Meredith	American Actor	Bipolar
George Michael	British Singer	Depression
Dimitri Mihalas	American Astronomer	Bipolar
Kate Millett	American Feminist Writer	Bipolar
Spike Milligan	Irish Comedian	Bipolar

Name	Prominence	Diagnosis
Claude Monet	French Artist	Depression
J. P. Morgan	American Financier	Bipolar
Alanis Morissette	Canadian Singer	Depression
Steven Patrick Morrissey	British Singer	Depression
Wolfgang Amadeus Mozart	Viennese Composer	Depression
John Mulheren	American Financier	Bipolar
Edvard Munch	Norwegian Artist	Depression
Robert Munsch	Canadian Writer	Bipolar
Ilie Nastase	Romanian Tennis Player	Bipolar
Willie Nelson	American Singer	Depression
Isaac Newton	British Physicist	Bipolar
Stevie Nicks	American Singer	Depression
Florence Nightingale	British Nurse	Bipolar
Gena Lee Nolin	American Actor	Postpartum
Deborah Norville	American Journalist	Depression
Graeme O'Bree	Scottish Cyclist	Depression
Sinead O'Connor	Irish Singer	Bipolar
Rosie O'Donnell	American Comedian	Depression
Georgia O'Keeffe	American Painter	Depression
Eugene O'Neill	American Playwright	Depression
Donny Osmond	American Singer	Depression
Marie Osmond	American Singer	Postpartum
Ronnie O'Sullivan	British Snooker Player	Bipolar
Gwyneth Paltrow	American Actor	Postpartum
Joe Pantoliano	American Actor	Depression
Charles Parker	American Jazz Composer	Depression
Dorothy Parker	American Writer	Depression
Dolly Parton	American Singer	Depression
George S. Patton	American General	Depression
Jane Pauley	American Journalist	Bipolar
Amanda Peet	American Actor	Postpartum
Pierre Péladeau	Canadian Publisher	Bipolar
Charley Pell	American Football Coach	Depression
Walker Percy	American Writer	Depression

Name	Prominence	Diagnosis
Murray Pezim	Canadian Financier	Bipolar
Mackenzie Phillips	American Actress	Depression
Kellie Pickler	American Singer	Depression
Chonda Pierce	American Comedian	Depression
Jimmy Piersall	American Baseball Player	Bipolar
Valerie Plame	American CIA Agent	Postpartum
Edgar Allan Poe	American Writer	Bipolar
Jackson Pollock	American Painter	Depression
Cole Porter	American Composer	Depression
Alma Powell	Wife of U.S. Secretary of State	Depression
Susan Powter	American Motivational Speaker	Depression
Charley Pride	American Singer	Depression
Queen Latifah	American Singer	Depression
Queen Victoria	Queen of Britain	Depression
Sergei Rachmaninoff	Russian Composer	Depression
Mac Rebenack (Dr. John)	American Singer	Bipolar
Lou Reed	American Singer	Depression
Jerry Remy	American Sports Broadcaster	Depression
Burt Reynolds	American Actor	Depression
Anne Rice	American Writer	Depression
Lisa Rinna	American Actor	Postpartum
Joan Rivers	American Comedian	Depression
Lynn Rivers	American Congresswoman	Bipolar
Barret Robbins	American Football Player	Bipolar
Paul Robeson	American Actor	Depression
Norman Rockwell	American Artist	Depression
Lyndsey Rodrigues	Australian TV Presenter	Depression
Peter Mark Roget	Creator of Thesaurus	Depression
Theodore Roosevelt	American President	Bipolar
Roseanne	American Comedian	Depression
Raymond Roussin	Archbishop for Diocese of Vancouver	Depression

Name	Prominence	Diagnosis
J. K. Rowling	British Writer	Depression
Winona Ryder	American Actor	Depression
Yves Saint Laurent	French Fashion Designer	Depression
Charles Schulz	American Cartoonist	Depression
Robert Schuman	German Composer	Bipolar
Jim Shea	American Olympic Skeleton Racer	Depression
Mary Shelley	British Writer	Depression
Brooke Shields	American Actor	Postpartum
Neil Simon	American Playwright	Depression
Paul Simon	American Singer	Depression
Lauren Slater	American Psychologist	Depression
Michael Slater	Australian Cricketer	Depression
Tony Slattery	British Comedian	Bipolar
Joey Slinger	Canadian Journalist	Depression
Tim Smith	Australian Rugby Player	Bipolar
Alonzo Spellman	American Football Player	Depression
Diana Spencer	Princess of Wales	Depression
Muffin Spencer-Devlin	American Golfer	Bipolar
Rick Springfield	Australian Actor/Singer	Depression
Bruce Springsteen	American Musician	Depression
Rod Steiger	American Actor	Depression
John Steinbeck	American Writer	Depression
George Stephanopoulos	American Political Analyst	Depression
Ben Stiller	American Actor	Bipolar
Sting	British Musician	Depression
Darryl Strawberry	American Baseball Player	Bipolar
Picabo Street	American Olympic Skier	Depression
William Styron	American Writer	Depression
Donna Summer	American Singer	Depression
Donald Sutherland	Canadian Actor	Depression
Shaun Tait	Australian Cricketer	Depression
Amy Tam	American Writer	Depression
James Taylor	American Musician	Depression

Name	Prominence	Diagnosis
Lili Taylor	American Actor	Bipolar
Nikki Teasley	American Basketball Player	Depression
Nikola Tesla	Austrian/American Inventor	Depression
Dylan Thomas	Welsh Poet	Depression
Emma Thompson	British Actor	Depression
Tracy Thompson	American Journalist	Depression
Gene Tierney	American Actor	Depression
Leo Tolstoy	Russian Writer	Depression
Henri de Toulouse-Lautrec	French Artist	Depression
Spencer Tracy	American Actor	Depression
Marcus Trescothick	British Cricket Player	Depression
Margaret Trudeau	Wife of Prime Minister (Canada)	Bipolar
Ted Turner	American Entrepreneur	Bipolar
Mark Twain	American Writer	Depression
Mike Tyson	American Boxer	Depression
Tracy Ullman	British Comedian	Bipolar
Dimitrius Underwood	American Football Player	Depression
Vivian Vance	American Actor	Depression
Jean-Claude Van Damme	Belgian Actor	Bipolar
Towns Van Zandt	American Musician	Bipolar
Ben Vereen	American Actor	Depression
Meredith Vieira	American Journalist	Depression
Lindsey Vonn	American Olympic Skier	Depression
Kurt Vonnegut	American Writer	Depression
Lars von Trier	Danish Film Director	Depression
Tom Waits	American Musician	Bipolar
Mike Wallace	American Journalist	Depression
David Walliams	British Comedian	Depression
Arthur Evelyn Waugh	British Writer	Depression
Damon Wayans	American Comedian	Depression
Mary Foresberg Weiland	American Model	Bipolar
Pete Wentz	American Musician	Bipolar
Robin Williams	American Comedian/Actor	Bipolar

Name	Prominence	Diagnosis
Serena Williams	American Tennis Player	Depression
Tennessee Williams	American Playwright	Depression
Brian Wilson	American Musician	Bipolar
Carnie Wilson	American Singer	Postpartum
Woodrow Wilson	American President	Depression
Oprah Winfrey	American Talk Show Host	Depression
Jonathan Winters	American Comedian	Bipolar
Frank Lloyd Wright	American Architect	Bipolar
Tammy Wynette	American Singer	Depression
Bert Yancey	American Golfer	Bipolar
Boris Yeltsin	President of Russian Federation	Depression
Robert Young	American Actor	Depression
Catherine Zeta-Jones	Welsh Actor	Bipolar
Warren Zevon	American Musician	Depression

Appendix C

Resources

ANTIBULLYING RESOURCES

Anti-Bully Training Centre
Website: antibullying.net

Anti-Defamation League
Website: adl.org/education/cyberbullying

Beat Bullying
Website: beatbullying.org

Cyberbullying National Prevention Crime Council
Website: ncpc.org/cyberbullying

Gay, Lesbian, and Straight Network
Website: glsen.org

It Gets Better
Website: itgetsbetter.org

National Bullying Prevention Center
Website: pacer.org/bullying

Stomp Out Bullying
Website: stompoutbullying.org

Stop Bullying
Website: stopbullying.gov

DEPRESSION AND BIPOLAR RESOURCES

Black Dog Institute—Australia
Website: blackdoginstitute.org.au

Blueprint for Hope—United States
Website: centerforloss.com

Child Adolescent Bipolar Foundation—United States
Website: bpkids.org

Child Mind Institute—United States
Website: childmind.org

Depression Alliance—United Kingdom
Website: depressionalliance.org

Depression and Bipolar Support Alliance—United States
Website: dbsalliance.org

Families for Depression Awareness—United States
Website: familyaware.org

International Foundation for Research and Education on Depression
Website: ifred.org

Mood Disorders Association of British Columbia—Canada
Website: www.mdabc.net

Mood Disorders Society of Canada
Website: mooddisorderscanada.ca

National Alliance on Mental Illness—United States
Website: nami.org

National Association for Research on Schizophrenia and Depression—
    United States
Website: narsad.org

National Network of Depression Centers—United States
Website: nndc.org

Seasonal Affective Disorder—United Kingdom
Website: sada.org.uk

GRIEF RESOURCES

Australian Centre for Grief and Bereavement
Website: grief.org.au

GriefShare—Canada
Website: griefshare.org

The Moyer Foundation—United States
Website: moyerfoundation.org/nbrg

The National Alliance for Grieving Children—United States
Website: childrengrieve.org

The National Center for Grieving Children & Families
Website: dougy.org

Rainbows International Grief Support for Children
Website: rainbows.org

MENTAL HEALTH ASSOCIATIONS

Canada
Canadian Mental Health Association
Website: cmha.ca

Europe
Mental Health Europe
Website: mhe-sme.org

South Africa
South African Federation for Mental Health
Website: safmh.org

United Kingdom
Mental Health Foundation
Website: mentalhealth.org.uk

United States
National Alliance on Mental Illness
Website: nami.org

National Institute of Mental Health
Website: nimh.nih.gov

National Mental Health Association
Website: nmha.org

Substance Abuse and Mental Health Services Administration
Website: samhsa.gov

World Association for Infant Mental Health
Website: waimh.org

PARENTING BOOKS

Engber, Andrea, and Leah Klungness. *The Complete Single Mother: Reassuring Answers to Your Most Challenging Concerns.* Avon: Adams Media, 2006.

Nadworny, John, and Cynthia Haddad. *The Special Needs Planning Guide: How to Prepare for Every Stage in Your Child's Life.* Baltimore: Brooks Publishing, 2007.

Phagan-Hansel, Kim. *The Foster Parent Toolbox.* Warren: EMK Press, 2012.

Schooler, Jayne, Thomas Atwood, and Bob Beltz. *The Whole Life Adoption Book: Realistic Advice for Building a Healthy Adoptive Family.* Colorado Springs: NavPress, 2008.

Shimberg, Elaine Fantle, and Michael Shimberg. *The Complete Single Father: Reassuring Answers to Your Most Challenging Concerns.* Avon: Adams Media, 2007.

PARENTING RESOURCES

Federation for Families for Children Mental Health
Website: ffcmh.org

Healthy Child Care America
Website: healthychildcare.org

National Foster Parent Organization
Website: nfpaonline.org

National Parent Help Line
Website: nationalparenthelpline.org

National Parent Teacher Association
Website: pta.org

National Parenting Education Network
Website: npen.org

One Tough Job
Website: onetoughjob.org

Parenting Resources
Website: usa.gov/Topics/Parents.shtml

Parents Advocating for Safe Schools
Website: parentsadvocatingforsafeschools.webs.com

Parents, Families, and Friends of Lesbians and Gays (PFLAG)
Website: community.pflag.org

PRESCRIPTION ASSISTANCE

Drug Card America
Website: drugcardamerica.com

Partnership for Prescription Assistance—United States
Website: pparx.org

Patient Assistance—United States
Website: patientassistance.com

Rx Assist—United States
Website: rxassist.org

SELF-HARM RESOURCES

The American Self-Harm Information Clearinghouse
Website: selfinjury.org

Cornell Research Program on Self-Injurious Behavior
Website: crpsib.com

Harmless—United Kingdom
Website: harmless.org.uk

Reach Out—Australia
Website: au.reachout.com/What-is-self-harm

Self-Injury Foundation—United States
Website: selfinjuryfoundation.org

Self-Injury Outreach and Support
Website: sioutreach.org

The Sidran Institute—United States
Website: sidran.org

To Write Love on Her Arms
Website: twloha.com

STIGMA RESOURCES

BASTA—The Alliance for Mentally Ill People—Germany
Website: openthedoors.de

Breaking the Silence—United States
Website: btslessonplans.org

BringChange2Mind—United States
Website: bringchange2mind.org

The Carter Center—United States
Website: cartercenter.org

Mental Illness Watch—United States
Website: miwatch.org

Mind—United Kingdom
Website: mind.org.uk

National Alliance on Mental Illness—United States
Website: nami.org

National Consortium on Stigma Empowerment—United States
Website: stigmaandempowerment.org

National Mental Health Clearinghouse—United States
Website: mhselfhelp.org

No Kidding? Me Too!—United States
Website: NoKiddingMeToo.org

SANE—Australia
Website: sane.org

SHIFT—United Kingdom
Website: www.shift.org.uk

Stamp Out Stigma—United Kingdom
Website: www.stampoutstigma.net

SUICIDE HOTLINES
National Suicide Prevention Hotline United States
T: 800-273-TALK (800-273-8255)
Website: suicidepreventionlifeline.org

R U OK?—Australia
T: 1800 629 354
Website: ruokday.com

Samaritans—Australia
T: 03 63 31 3355
Website: samaritans.org

Samaritans—Ireland
T: (Ireland) 1850 60 90 90
Website: samaritans.org

Samaritans—United Kingdom
T: (United Kingdom) +44 (0) 8457 90 90 90
Website: samaritans.org

Samaritans—United States
T: 877-870-HOPE (877-870-4673)
Website: samaritansusa.org

Suicide Action Montreal—Canada
T: 514-723-4000
Website: suicideactionmontreal.qc.ca

The Trevor Project
T: 866-4-U-TREVOR (866-488-7386)
Website: thetrevorproject.org

SUICIDE PREVENTION RESOURCES
American Association of Suicidology—United States
Website: suicidology.org

American Foundation for Suicide Prevention
Website: afsp.org

Centers for Disease Control and Prevention, National Center for Injury
    Prevention and Control—United States
Website: cdc.gov/ncipc

Centre for Suicide Prevention—Canada
Website: suicideinfo.ca

Hopeline
Website: hopeline.com

International Association for Suicide Prevention—Norway
Website: iasp.info

Suicide Prevention Action Network—United States
Website: spanusa.org

Suicide Prevention Initiatives
Website: spiorg.org

Notes

CHAPTER 1. UNDERSTANDING CHILD DEVELOPMENT

1. A. A. Milne and Ernest Shepard, *Winnie-the-Pooh* (New York: Dutton, 1988).

2. Merriam Webster, *Merriam Webster's Collegiate Dictionary* (Springfield: Merriam Webster Publishing, 2001).

3. Rosemarie Jarski, *Words from the Wise: Over 6,000 of the Smartest Things Ever Said* (New York: Skyhorse Publishing, 2007).

4. Ibid.

5. John Bates, "Applications of Temperament Concepts," in *Temperament in Childhood*, ed. Geldolph Kohnstamm, Mary Rothbart, and John Bates, 321–55 (New York: Wiley, 1989).

6. Kathleen Gallagher, "Does Child Temperament Moderate the Influence of Parenting on Adjustment?" *Developmental Review* 22 (2002): 623–43.

7. Alexander Thomas, Stella Chess, and H. G. Birch, *Temperament and Behavior Disorders in Children* (New York: New York University Press, 1968).

8. Maria Garstein, Samuel Putnam, and Mary Rothbart, "Etiology of Preschool Behavior Problems: Contributions of Temperament Attributes in Early Childhood," *Clinical Child and Adolescent Psychology* 33 (2004): 21–31.

9. Giampaolo Perna, Danila di Pasquale et al., "Temperament, Character, and Anxiety Sensitivity in Panic Disorder: A High Risk Study," *Psychopathology* 45 (2012): 300–304.

10. Bruce Compas, Jennifer Connor-Smith, and S. S. Jaser, "Temperament, Stress Reactivity, and Coping: Implications for Depression in Childhood and Adolescence," *Journal of Clinical Child and Adolescent Psychology* 33 (2004): 21–31.

11. Mary Rothbart, David E. Evans, and Stephan A. Ahadi, "Temperament and Personality: Origins and Outcomes," *Journal of Personality and Social Psychology* 78, no. 1 (2000): 122–35.

12. Ed Diener, "Subjective Well-Being: The Science of Happiness and a Proposal for a National Index," *American Psychologist* 55 (2000): 34–43.

13. World Health Organization, *Mental Health: New Understanding, New Hope. The World Health Report* (Geneva: World Health Organization, 2001).

CHAPTER 2. DEFINING DEPRESSION IN CHILDHOOD

1. Mick Power, *Mood Disorders: A Handbook of Science and Practice* (London: John Wiley & Sons, 2004).

2. Daniel Stein, David Kupfer, and Alan Schatzberg, *Textbook of Mood Disorders* (Arlington: American Psychiatric Association, 2003).

3. William Parry-Jones, "History of Child and Adolescent Psychiatry," in *Child and Adolescent Psychiatry: Modern Approaches*, ed. Michael Rutter, Lionel Hersov, and Eric Taylor, 794–812 (Oxford: Blackwell Scientific, 1993).

4. Stanley Jackson, *Melancholia and Depression: From Hippocratic Times to Modern Times* (New Haven, CT: Yale University Press, 1990).

5. Andreas Marneros and Frederick Goodwin, *Bipolar Disorders: Mixed States, Rapid Cycling, and Atypical Forms* (New York: Cambridge University Press, 2005).

6. Jennifer Radden, *The Nature of Melancholy: From Aristotle to Kristeva* (New York: Oxford University Press, 2002).

7. Ian Gotlib and Constance Hammen, *Handbook of Depression* (New York: Guilford Press, 2009).

8. Joan Luby et al., "Preschool Major Depressive Disorder: Preliminary Validation for Developmentally Modified DSM-IV Criteria," *Journal of the American Academy of Child and Adolescent Psychiatry* 41 (2002): 928–37.

9. Gregory Miller and Steve Cole, "Clustering of Depression and Inflammation in Adolescents Previously Exposed to Childhood Adversity," *Biological Psychiatry* 72 (2012): 34–40.

10. David Cole et al., "A Longitudinal Study of Cognitive Risks for Depressive Symptoms in Children and Young Adolescents," *Journal of Early Adolescence* 31 (2012): 782–16.

11. Kathleen Merikangas et al., "The National Comorbidity Survey Adolescent Supplement (NCS-A): I. Background and Measures," *Journal of the American Academy of Child Adolescent Psychiatry* 48 (2009): 367–69; National Institute of Mental Health, "Major Depressive Disorder in Children," National Institute of Mental Health, http://www.nimh.nih.gov/statistics/1mdd_child.shtml (accessed January 31, 2013).

12. G. Zalsman et al., "Neurobiology of Depression in Children and Adolescents," *Child and Adolescent Psychiatric Clinics of North America* 15 (2006): 843–68.

13. Joel Nigg, "Temperament and Developmental Psychopathology," *Journal of Child Psychology and Psychiatric and Allied Disciplines* 47 (2006): 395–422.

14. S. E. Gilman et al., "Socio-Economic Status, Family Disruption, and Residential Stability in Childhood: Relation to Onset, Recurrence, and Remission of Major Depression," *Psychological Medicine* 33 (2003): 1341–55.

15. Sheryl Goodman and Ian Gotlib, "Risk for Psychopathology in Children of Depressed Mothers: A Developmental Model for Understanding Mechanisms of Transmission," *Psychological Review* 106 (1999): 458–90.

16. ABCNews.com, "One in 40 Infants Experience Baby Blues, Doctors Say," November 9, 2009, http://abcnews.go.com/Health/OnCall/story?id=2640591&page=1 (accessed January 25, 2013).

17. Zero to Three, *Diagnostic Classification of Mental Health and Developmental Disorders of Infancy and Early Childhood*, revised edition (Washington, DC: Zero to Three Press, 2005).

18. Joan Luby et al., "The Clinical Significance of Preschool Depression: Impairment in Functioning and Clinical Markers of the Disorder," *Journal of Affective Disorders* 112 (2009): 111–19.

19. Thomas Delate et al., "Trends in the Use of Antidepressants in a National Sample of Uninsured Pediatric Patients, 1988 to 2002," *Psychiatric Services* 55 (2004): 387–91.

20. Renee Thompson and Howard Berenbaum, "Shame Reactions to Everyday Dilemmas Are Associated with Depressive Disorder," *Cognitive Therapy and Research* 30 (2006): 415–25.

21. Joan Luby et al., "The Clinical Picture of Depression in Preschool Children," *Journal of the American Academy of Child and Adolescent Psychiatry* 42 (2003): 340–48.

22. Rita Wicks-Nelson and Allen Israel, *Abnormal Child and Adolescent Psychology* (Upper Saddle River, NJ: Pearson, 2009).

23. Janet Kistner et al., "Helplessness in Early Childhood: Prediction of Symptoms Associated with Depression and Negative Self-Worth," *Merrill-Palmer Quarterly* 47 (2001): 336–41; Gabrielle Carlson, "The Challenge of Diagnosing Depression in Childhood and Adolescence," *Journal of Affective Disorders* 61 (2003): 3–8.

24. Jarad Kashani et al., "Developmental Perspectives in Child and Adolescent Depressive Symptoms in a Community Sample," *American Journal of Psychiatry* 146 (1989): 871–75.

25. Harold Koplewicz, *More Than Moody: Recognizing and Treating Adolescent Depression* (New York: GP Putnam, 2003).

26. Substance Abuse and Mental Health Services Administration, "Depression Rates Triple between the Ages of 12 and 15 Among Adolescent Girls," July 24, 2012, http://www.samhsa.gov/newsroom/advisories/1207241656.aspx (accessed April 10, 2013).

27. Deborah Serani, *Living with Depression* (Lanham, MD: Rowman & Littlefield, 2011).

28. Mauro Garcia-Toro and Iratxe Aguirre, "Biopsychosocial Model in Depression Revisited," *Medical Hypotheses* 68 (2007): 683–91.

29. Gotlib and Hammen, *Handbook of Depression.*

CHAPTER 3. DIAGNOSING PEDIATRIC DEPRESSION

1. Jack Shonkoff and Deborah Phillips, *From Neurons to Neighborhoods: The Science of Early Childhood Development* (Washington, DC: National Academies Press, 2000).

2. Ibid.

3. Helen Egger and Robert Emde, "Developmentally Sensitive Diagnostic Criteria for Mental Health Disorders in Early Childhood," *American Psychologist* 66 (2011): 95–106.

4. Stanley Greenspan and Serena Weider, *Infant and Early Childhood Mental Health: A Comprehensive Developmental Approach to Assessment* (Arlington: American Psychiatric Association, 2005).

5. Aaron Beck et al., *Manual for the Beck Depression Inventory-II* (San Antonio: Psychological Corporation, 1996).

6. Maria Kovacs, *The Children's Depression Inventory* (North Tonawanda, NY: Multi-Health Systems, 1992).

7. Keith Conners, *Conners Comprehensive Behavior Rating Scales* (Austin: Pro-Ed, 2008).

8. Georgia DeGangi et al., *Infant/Toddler Symptom Checklist: A Screening Tool for Parents* (San Antonio: Psychological Corporation, 1995).

9. Nadine Melhem et al., "Phenomenology and Correlates of Complicated Grief in Children and Adolescents," *Journal of the American Academy of Child and Adolescent Psychiatry* 46 (2007): 493–99.

10. Theodore Millon and Carrie Millon, *Manual for the Millon Adolescent Clinical Inventory* (Minneapolis: National Computer Systems, 2006).

11. Conway F. Saylor et al., "The Pediatric Emotional Distress Scale: A Brief Screening Measure for Young Children Exposed to Traumatic Events," *Journal of Clinical Child Psychology* 28 (1999): 70–81.

12. William Reynolds, *Reynolds Adolescent Depression Scale, 2nd edition: Short Form* (Lutz, FL: Psychological Assessment Resources, 2008).

13. William Reynolds, *Reynolds Child Depression Scale—2* (Lutz, FL: Psychological Assessment Resources, 2010).

14. John Briere, *Trauma Symptom Checklist for Young Children: Professional Manual* (Odessa: Psychological Assessment Resources, 2005).

15. American Psychiatric Association, *Diagnostic and Statistical Manual of Mental Disorders*, 5th edition (Washington, DC: American Psychiatric Association, 2013).

16. Zero to Three, *Diagnostic Classification of Mental Health and Developmental Disorders of Infancy and Early Childhood*, revised edition (Washington, DC: Zero to Three Press, 2005).

17. World Health Organization, *International Statistical Classification of Diseases and Related Health Problems*, 10th revision (Geneva: World Health Organization Press, 2004).

18. Shashi Bhatia and Subhash Bhatia, "Childhood and Adolescent Depression," *American Family Physician* 75 (2007): 73–80.

19. American Psychiatric Association, *Diagnostic and Statistical Manual of Mental Disorders*.

20. Norman Rosenthal, *Winter Blues: Everything You Need to Know to Beat Seasonal Affective Disorder*, revised edition (New York: Guilford Press, 2005).

21. Maria Kovacs et al., "Childhood-Onset Dysthymic Disorder: Clinical Features and Prospective Naturalistic Outcome," *Archives of General Psychiatry* 51 (1994): 365–74.

22. Bhatia and Bhatia, "Childhood and Adolescent Depression."

23. Lydia Gries, "Adjustment Disorder Related to Bereavement," *Journal for Nurse Practitioners* 8 (2012): 186–94.

24. Julie Kaplow et al., "DSM-V Diagnostic Criteria for Bereavement-Related Disorders in Children and Adolescents: Developmental Considerations," *Psychiatry* 75 (2012): 243–66.

25. Boris Birmaher et al., "Childhood and Adolescent Depression: A Review of the Past 10 Years. Part I," *Journal of the American Academy of Child and Adolescent Psychiatry* 35 (1996): 1427–39.

26. Hagop Akiskal, "Dysthymia and Cyclothymia in Psychiatric Practice a Century after Kraepelin," *Journal of Affective Disorders* 62 (2001): 17–31.

27. Julie Faste and John Preston, *Taking Charge of Bipolar Disorder* (New York: Hachette Group, 2006).

28. Petronella Vant Veer-Tazelaar et al., "Stepped-Care Prevention of Anxiety and Depression in Late Life: A Randomized Controlled Trial," *Archives of General Psychiatry* 66 (2009): 297–304.

29. William Beardslee and Tracy Gladstone, "Prevention of Childhood Depression: Recent Findings and Future Prospects," *Biological Psychiatry* 49 (2001): 1101–10.

CHAPTER 4. TREATMENTS FOR PEDIATRIC DEPRESSION

1. Nadine Kaslow et al., "Family Based Interventions for Child and Adolescent Disorders," *Journal of Marital and Family Therapy* 38 (2012): 82–100.

2. Karen Kasch et al., "Behavioral Activation and Inhibition Systems and the Severity and Course of Depression," *Journal of Abnormal Psychology* 111 (2002): 589–97.

3. Chrissie Verduyn, Julia Rogers, and Alison Wood, *Depression: Cognitive Behavioral Therapy with Children and Young People* (London: Routledge, 2009).

4. Tina Goldstein et al., "Dialectical Behavior Therapy for Adolescents with Bipolar Disorder: A 1-Year Open Trial," *Journal of the American Academy of Child Adolescent Psychiatry* 46 (2007): 820–30.

5. Miles Thompson and Jeremy Gauntlett-Gilbert, "Mindfulness with Children and Adolescents: Effective Clinical Application," *Clinical Child Psychology & Psychiatry* 13 (2008): 395–407.

6. Shannon Lenze, Jennifer Pautsch, and Joan Luby, "Parent-Child Interaction Therapy Emotion Development: A Novel Treatment for Depression in Preschool Children," *Depression and Anxiety* 28 (2011): 153–59.

7. Sue Bratton et al., "The Efficacy of Play Therapy with Children: A Meta-Analytic Review of Treatment Outcomes," *Professional Psychology: Research and Practice* 36 (2005): 376–90.

8. Charles Schaefer, *Foundations of Play Therapy* (New York: John Wiley & Sons, 2011).

9. Hildegard Horn et al., "Efficacy of Psychodynamic Short-Term Psychotherapy for Children and Adolescents with Depression," *Praxis der Kinderpsychologie & Kinderpsychiatrie* 54 (2005): 578–97.

10. Marshall Becker and Lois Maiman, "Sociobehavioral Determinants of Compliance with Health and Medical Care Recommendations," *Medical Care* 13 (1975): 10–24.

11. Fadi Maalouf, Mia Atwi, and David Brent, "Treatment-Resistant Depression in Adolescents: Review and Updates on Clinical Management," *Depression and Anxiety* 28 (2011): 946–54.

12. Neer Ghaziuddin et al., "Practice Parameter for Use of Electroconvulsive Therapy with Adolescents," *Journal of the American Academy of Child and Adolescent Psychiatry* 43 (2004): 1521–39.

13. Yuval Bloch et al., "Repetitive Transcranial Magnetic Stimulation in the Treatment of Depression in Adolescents: An Open-Label Study," *Journal of ECT* 24 (2008): 156–59.

14. Z. J. Yu et al., "Vagus Nerve Stimulation: Can It Be Used in Adolescents or Children with Treatment Resistant Depression?" *Current Psychiatry* 10 (2008): 116–22.

15. Pierre Blier, Daniel Zigman, and Jean Blier, "On the Safety and Benefits of Repeated Intravenous Injections of Ketamine for Depression," *Biological Psychiatry* 72 (2012): e11–12.

16. Andre Brunoni et al., "The Sertraline vs. Electrical Current Therapy for Treating Depression Clinical Study," *JAMA Psychiatry* 1 (2013): 1–9.

17. G. C. Albert et al., "Deep Brain Stimulation, Vagal Nerve Stimulation, and Transcranial Stimulation: An Overview of Stimulation Parameters and Neurotransmitter Release," *Neuroscience & Biobehavioral Reviews* 37 (2009): 1042–60.

18. Lawrence Lesko, "Personalized Medicine: Elusive Dream or Imminent Reality?" *Clinical Pharmacology & Therapeutics* 81 (2005): 807–16.

CHAPTER 5. HOLISTIC APPROACHES TO DEPRESSION

1. Jon Kabat-Zinn, *Coming to Our Senses: Healing Ourselves and the World through Mindfulness* (New York: Hyperion, 2011).

2. David Sousa, *How the Brain Learns* (Thousand Oaks, CA: Sage Publications, 2006).

3. Shawn Smith, *The User's Guide to the Human Mind: Why Our Brains Make Us Unhappy, Anxious, and Neurotic and What We Can Do About It* (Oakland: New Harbinger Publications, 2011).

4. Kabat-Zinn, *Coming to Our Senses.*

5. Stephen Kaplan, "The Restorative Benefits of Nature: Toward an Integrative Framework," *Journal of Environmental Psychology* 15 (1995): 169–82.

6. Samina Azeemi et al., "A Critical Analysis of Chromotherapy and Its Scientific Evolution," *Evidence-Based Complementary and Alternative Medicine* 2 (2005): 481–88.

7. Robin McKie, "Mood Lighting Used to Boost Pupil's Academic Performance at Surrey School," *The Guardian*, April 30, 2011, http://www.guardian.co.uk/education/2011/may/01/mood-lighting-boost-academic-performance (accessed November 15, 2012).

8. Peter Barrett and Lucinda Barrett, "The Potential of Positive Places: Senses, Rain, and Spaces," *Intelligent Buildings International* 2 (2010): 46–52.

9. Anthony Synnott, "Roses, Coffee, and Lovers: The Meanings of Smell," *Compendium of Olfactory Research* 19 (1994): 117–28.

10. Judith White, *Aromatherapy for Men* (Bloomington: Balboa Press, 2011).

11. Catherine Harmer et al., "Negative Ion Treatment Increases Positive Emotional Processing in Seasonal Affective Disorder," *Psychological Medicine* 42 (2011): 1605–12.

12. Pierce Howard, *The Owner's Manual for the Brain: Everyday Applications from Mind-Brain Research* (Austin: Bard Press, 2006); Michael Terman and Jiuan Su Terman, "Treatment of Seasonal Affective Disorder with a High-Output Negative Ionizer," *Journal of Alternative and Complementary Medicine* 1 (1995): 87–92.

13. Jolanda Mass et al., "Morbidity Is Related to a Green Living Environment," *Journal of Epidemiology and Community Health* 63 (2009): 967–73.

14. Catherine Rice-Evans and Lester Packer, *Flavonoids in Health and Disease* (New York: Marcel Dekker, 2003).

15. Betsy Hornick and Roberta Larson Duyff, *American Dietetic Association: Complete Food & Nutrition Guide* (Hoboken, NJ: John Wiley & Sons, 2012).

16. Kelly Shaw, Jane Turner, and Chris Del Mar, "Tryptophan and 5-Hydroxytryptophan for Depression," *Cochrane Database of Systematic Reviews* 4 (2003): Cd003198.

17. Carolyn Dean, *The Miracle of Magnesium* (New York: Ballantine, 2006).

18. Joseph Hibbeln, "Fish Consumption and Major Depression," *Lancet* 351 (1998): 1213.

19. Hanah Nemets et al., "Omega-3 Treatment of Childhood Depression: A Controlled, Double-Blind Pilot Study," *American Journal of Psychiatry* 163 (2006): 1098–1100.

20. Patrick Holdford, "Depression: The Nutrition Connection," *Primary Care Mental Health* 1 (2003): 9–16.

21. Yong-Ku Kim et al., "Differences in Cytokines between Non-Suicidal Patients and Suicidal Patients in Major Depression," *Progress in Neuro-Psychopharmacology and Biological Psychiatry* 15 (2008): 356–61.

22. Goren Högberg et al., "Depressed Adolescents in a Case-Series Were Low in Vitamin D and Depression Was Ameliorated by Vitamin D Supplementation," *Acta Paediatrica* 101 (2012): 779–83.

23. James Dowds and Diane Stafford, *The Vitamin D Cure* (Hoboken, NJ: John Wiley & Sons, 2012).

24. Fernando Gómez-Pinilla, "Brain Foods: The Effects of Nutrients on Brain Functioning," *Nature Reviews Neuroscience* 9 (2008): 568–78.

25. Kai MacDonald and Tina Marie MacDonald, "The Peptide That Binds: A Systematic Review of Oxytocin and Its Prosocial Effects in Humans," *Harvard Review of Psychiatry* 18 (2012): 39–52.

26. Thomas Insel and Larry Young, "The Neurobiology of Attachment," *National Review of Neuroscience* 2 (2001): 129–36.

27. Wayne Drevets, "Orbitofrontal Cortex Function and Structure of Depression," *Annals of the New York Academy of Sciences* 1121 (2007): 499–527.

28. Denise Adams et al., "The Safety of Pediatric Acupuncture: A Systematic Review," *Pediatrics* 128 (2011): 1011–91.

29. Ibid.

30. Raphael Leo and Jesus Salvador Ligot, "A Systematic Review of Randomized Controlled Trials of Acupuncture in the Treatment of Depression," *Journal of Affective Disorders* 97 (2007): 13–22.

31. Tiffany Field, "Exercise Research on Children and Adolescents," *Complementary Therapies in Clinical Practice* 18 (2000): 54–59.

32. Chanudda Nabkasorn et al., "Effects of Physical Exercise on Depression, Neuroendocrine Stress Hormones, and Physiological Fitness in Adolescent Females with Depressive Symptoms," *European Journal of Public Health* 16 (2006): 179–84.

33. Karen L. Hill, "Promoting Exercise Compliance: A Cognitive-Behavioral Approach," *Women and Therapy* 25 (2002): 75–90.

34. Marybetts Sinclair, *Pediatric Massage Therapy* (Philadelphia: Lippincott, Williams & Wilkins, 2004).

35. Lynea Gillen and James Gillen, *Yoga Calm for Children: Educating Heart, Mind, and Body* (Portland: Three Pebbles Press, 2007).

36. Mary Lou Galantino, Robyn Galbavy, and Lauren Quinn, "Therapeutic Effects of Yoga for Children: A Systematic Review of the Literature," *Pediatric Physical Therapy* 20 (2008): 66–80.

37. Paula Boyajian, "Yoga for the Child with Special Needs," *Exceptional Parent* 4 (2004): 28–30.

38. Ibid.

39. Tere Bowen-Irish, "Bringing Yoga into the Classroom: You'll Be Surprised at What It Does," *YogaKids International Articles* (2005): 418.

40. John Sloboda, "Empirical Studies of Emotional Response to Music," in *Cognitive Bases of Musical Communication*, ed. Mari Riess Jones and Susan Holleran, 33–46 (Washington, DC: American Psychological Association, 1991).

41. Patrik N. Juslin and John Sloboda, *Handbook of Music and Emotion: Theory, Research, and Applications* (New York: Oxford University Press, 2011).

42. John Sloboda, *Exploring the Musical Mind: Cognition, Emotions, Ability, Function* (New York: Oxford University Press, 2005).

43. Anna Milani, Marissa Lorusso, and Massimo Molteni, "The Effects of Audiobooks on the Psychosocial Adjustment of Pre-Adolescents and Adolescents with Dyslexia," *Dyslexia* 16 (2010): 87–97.

44. Elliott Salamon et al., "Sound Therapy Induced Relaxation: Down Regulating Stress Processes and Pathologies," *Medical Science Monitor* 9 (2003): RA96–RA101.

45. Byrd Baylor and Peter Parnall, *The Other Way to Listen* (New York: Simon & Schuster, 1978).

46. Anne LeClaire, *Listening Below the Noise: The Transformational Power of Silence* (New York: Harper Perennial, 2010).

47. Kathi Kemper, Sunita Vohra, and Richard Walls, "The Use of Complementary and Alternative Medicine in Pediatrics," *Pediatrics* 122 (2008): 1374–86.

48. Ruth Leyse-Wallace, *Linking Nutrition to Mental Health* (New York: iUniverse, 2008).

CHAPTER 6. SELF-HARM AND SUICIDE

1. Colleen Jacobson and Madelyn Gould, "The Epidemiology and Phenomenology of Non-Suicidal Self-Injurious Behavior among Adolescents: A Critical Review of the Literature," *Archives of Suicide Research* 11 (2007): 129–47.

2. Centers for Disease Control and Prevention, "CDC Wonder Database: Mortality Query," Centers for Disease Control, http://wonder.cdc.gov (accessed February 17, 2013).

3. Yu Jin Lee et al., "Direct and Indirect Effects of the Temperament and Character on Alexithymia: A Pathway Analysis with Mood and Anxiety," *Comprehensive Psychiatry* 51 (2010): 201–6.

4. Margaret Andover and Brandon Gibb, "Non-Suicidal Self-Injury, Attempted Suicide, and Suicidal Intent among Psychiatric Inpatients," *Psychiatry Research* 178 (2010): 101–5.

5. Rendueles Villalba and Colin J. Harrington, "Repetitive Self-Injurious Behavior: A Neuropsychiatric Perspective and Review of Pharmacologic Treatments," *Seminars in Clinical Neuropsychiatry* 5 (2000): 215–26.

6. Richard J. Bodnar, "Neuropharmacological and Neuroendocrine Substrates of Stress-Induced Analgesia," *Annals of the New York Academy of Science* 467 (1986): 345–60.

7. Deborah Serani, *Living with Depression* (Lanham, MD: Rowman & Littlefield, 2011).

8. Victoria E. White Kress, "Self-Injurious Behaviors: Assessment and Diagnosis," *Journal of Counseling and Development* 81 (2003): 490–96.

9. Ibid.

10. Pamela J. Dieter et al., "Self-Injury and Self-Capacities: Assisting an Individual in Crisis," *Journal of Clinical Psychology* 56 (2000): 1173–91.

11. Tim Dalgleish et al., "Method-of-Loci as a Mnemonic Device to Facilitate Access to Self-Affirming Personal Memories for Individuals with Depression," *Clinical Psychological Science* (2013), in press.

12. Steven Levenkron, *Cutting: Understanding and Overcoming Self-Mutilation* (New York: W. W. Norton, 1999).

13. Madelyn Gould et al., "Youth Suicide Risk and Preventive Interventions: A Review of the Past 10 Years," *Journal of the American Academy of Child and Adolescent Psychiatry* 42 (2003): 386–405.

14. Centers for Disease Control and Prevention, "Youth Suicide and Attempted Suicide," *Morbidity and Mortality Weekly Report* 53 (2004): 471.

15. M. David Rudd et al., "Warning Signs for Suicide: Theory, Research, and Clinical Applications," *Suicide and Life-Threatening Behavior* 36 (2006): 255–62; U.S. Preventive Services Task Force, "Screening for Suicide Risk: Recommendation and Rationale," *Annals of Internal Medicine* 140 (2004): 820–21.

16. Lucy Davidson and Markku Linnoila, *Risk Factors for Youth Suicide* (New York: Taylor & Francis Group, 1990).

17. Kelly Posner et al., "Columbia Classification Algorithm of Suicide Assessment: Classification of Suicidal Events in the FDA's Pediatric Suicidal Risk Analysis of Antidepressants," *American Journal of Psychiatry* 164 (2007): 1035–43.

18. Tamar Lasky et. al., "Children's Hospitalizations with a Mood Disorder Diagnosis in General Hospitals in the United States 2000–2006," *Child and Adolescent Psychiatry and Mental Health* 5 (2011): 27–36.

CHAPTER 7. MY CHILD IS DIAGNOSED, NOW WHAT?

1. Pamela Wilansky-Traynor et al., "Cognitive Behavioural Therapy for Depressed Youth: Predictors of Attendance in a Pilot Study," *Journal of the Canadian Academy of Child and Adolescent Psychiatry* 19 (2010): 81–87.

2. Amy Shuman and Jeremy P. Shapiro, "The Effects of Preparing Parents for Child Psychotherapy on Accuracy of Expectations and Treatment Attendance," *Community Mental Health Journal* 38 (2002): 3–16.

3. Miron Zuckerman et al., "On the Importance of Self-Determination for Intrinsically Motivated Behavior," *Personality and Social Psychology Bulletin* 4 (1978): 443–46.

4. Helen Lazaratou et al., "Parental Attitudes and Opinions on the Use of Psychotropic Medication in Mental Disorders of Childhood," *Annals of General Psychiatry* 6 (2007): 1–7.

5. Jack Stevens et al., "Parental Attitudes toward Children's Use of Antidepressants and Psychotherapy," *Journal of Child and Adolescent Psychopharmacology* 19 (2009): 289–96.

6. C. Steven Richards and Michael G. Perri, *Relapse Prevention for Depression* (Washington, DC: American Psychological Association, 2010).

7. P. K. Gillman, "Serotonin Syndrome: History and Risks," *Fundamental and Clinical Pharmacology* 12 (2009): 482–91.

8. Jonathan Price et al., "Emotional Side-Effects of Selective Serotonin Reuptake Inhibitors: Qualitative Study," *British Journal of Psychiatry* 195 (2009): 211–17.

9. Jeffrey A. Bridge, "Clinical Response and Risk for Reported Suicidal Ideation and Suicide Attempts in Pediatric Antidepressant Treatment: A Meta-Analysis of Randomized Controlled Trials," *Journal of the American Medical Association* 297 (2007): 1683–96.

10. John Curry et al., "Recovery and Recurrence Following Treatment for Adolescent Major Depression," *Archives of General Psychiatry* 68 (2011): 263–69.

11. National Institute of Mental Health, "Antidepressant Medications for Children and Adolescents: Information for Parents and Caregivers," National Institute of Mental Health, http://www.nimh.nih.gov/health/topics/child-and-adolescent-mental-health/antidepressant-medications-for-children-and-adolescents-information-for-parents-and-caregivers.shtml (accessed December 13, 2013).

12. U.S. Preventive Services Task Force, "Screening and Treatment for Major Depressive Disorder in Children and Adolescents: U.S. Preventive Services Task Force Recommendation Statement," *Pediatrics* 123 (2009): 1223–28.

13. Deborah Perlick et al., "Stigma as a Barrier to Recovery: Adverse Effects of Perceived Stigma on Social Adaptation of Persons Diagnosed with Bipolar Disorder," *Psychiatric Services* 52 (2001): 1627–31.

CHAPTER 8. TIPS FOR PARENTING YOUR DEPRESSED CHILD

1. National Alliance on Mental Illness, *A Family Guide: What Families Need to Know About Adolescent Depression* (Arlington: National Alliance on Mental Illness, 2011).

2. Jeffrey Miller, *The Childhood Depression Sourcebook* (New York: McGraw Hill, 1999).

3. J. David Hawkins et al., "Preventing Adolescent Health-Risk Behaviors by Strengthening Protection during Childhood," *Archives of Pediatric and Adolescent Medicine* 153 (1999): 226–34.

4. Ralph E. Cash, "When It Hurts to Be a Teenager," *Principal Leadership Magazine* 4 (2003): 1–6.

5. "Building the Legacy," IDEA Government, http://idea.ed.gov (accessed November 13, 2012).

6. Heather A. Turner and Paul A. Muller, "Long-Term Effects of Child Corporal Punishment on Depressive Symptoms in Young Adults: Potential Moderators and Mediators," *Journal of Family Issues* 25 (2004): 761–82.

7. Forrest S. Mosten, *Collaborative Divorce Handbook* (San Francisco: John Wiley & Sons, 2009).

8. Dan Kindlon, *Too Much of a Good Thing: Raising Children of Character in an Indulgent Age* (New York: Miramax Books, 2001).

9. Amy Mendenhall and Katherine Mount, "Parents of Children with Mental Illness: Exploring the Caregiver Experience and Caregiver-Focused Interventions," *Families in Society* 92 (2010): 183–90.

10. Julie Robison et al., "A Broader View of Family Caregiving: Effects of Caregiving and Caregiver Conditions on Depressive Symptoms, Health, Work, and Social Isolation," *Psychological Science* 64 (2009): 788–98.

11. National Marriage Project, "The Date Night Opportunity," National Marriage Project, http://nationalmarriageproject.org (accessed February 20, 2013).

CHAPTER 9. TWENTY DEPRESSION MYTHS EVERY PARENT SHOULD KNOW

1. Patrick Corrigan et al., "Stigmatizing Attitudes about Mental Illness and Allocation of Resources to Mental Health Services," *Community Mental Health Journal* 40 (2004): 297–307.

2. Norman Sartorius and Hugh Schulze, *Reducing the Stigma of Mental Illness: A Report from a Global Association* (London: Cambridge University Press, 2005).

3. Deborah Serani, *Living with Depression* (Lanham, MD: Rowman & Littlefield, 2011).

4. World Health Organization, *Integrating Mental Health into Primary Care: A Global Perspective* (Geneva: World Health Organization, 2008).

5. Patrick Corrigan and F. Miller, "Shame, Blame, and Contamination: A Review of the Impact of Mental Illness Stigma on Family Members," *Journal of Mental Health* 13 (2004): 537–48.

6. Otto Wahl, *Media Madness: Public Images of Mental Illness* (New Brunswick, NJ: Rutgers University Press, 1995); Andrea Lawson and Gregory Fouts, "Mental Illness in Disney Animated Films," *Canadian Journal of Psychiatry* 49 (2004): 310–14.

7. Patrick Corrigan and Ann Watson, "The Paradox of Self-Stigma and Mental Illness," *Clinical Psychology: Science and Practice* 9 (2002): 35–53.

8. J. K. Martin, "The Construction of Fear: Americans' Preferences for Social Distance from Children and Adolescents with Mental Health Problems," *Journal of Health and Social Behavior* 48 (2007): 50–67.

9. Peter Byrne, "Stigma of Mental Illness and Ways of Diminishing It," *Advances in Psychiatric Treatment* 6 (2000): 65–72.

10. Mark Schaller et al., *Evolution, Culture, and the Human Mind* (New York: Psychology Press, 2010).

11. E. Goffman, *Stigma: Notes on the Management of Spoiled Identity* (Englewood, NJ: Prentice-Hall, 1963).

CHAPTER 10. PLANNING FOR THE FUTURE

1. Simon Olshansky, "Chronic Sorrow: A Response to Having a Mentally Defective Child," *Social Casework* 43 (1962): 190–93.

2. Peggy MacGregor, "Grief: The Unrecognized Parental Response to Mental Illness in a Child," *Social Work* 39 (1994): 160–66.

3. William E. Narrow et al., "Mental Health Service Use by Americans with Severe Mental Illnesses," *Social of Psychiatry and Psychiatric Epidemiology* 35 (2000): 147–55.

4. Steven J. Bartels, "Caring for the Whole Person: Integrated Health Care for Older Adults with Severe Mental Illness and Medical Comorbidity," *Journal of the American Geriatric Society* 52 (2004): S249–57.

5. Mitzi Walsh, *Bipolar Disorders: A Guide to Helping Children and Adolescents* (Sebastopol: O'Reilly & Associates, 2000).

6. Deborah Elbaum, "Special Needs Care for Adult Children: Care Options," Care.com, http://www.care.com/special-needs-care-options-p1145-q5906.html (accessed March 1, 2013).

7. Mona Wasow, *The Skipping Stone: The Rippling Effect of Mental Illness in the Family* (Palo Alto, CA: Science and Behavior Books, 1995); Yvonne Darlington and Robert Bland, "Strategies for Encouraging and Maintaining Hope among People Living with Serious Mental Illness," *Australian Social Work* 52 (1999): 17–24.

Glossary

acoustic sound therapy: the use of soundscapes to enhance well-being.

adjustment disorder related to bereavement (ADRB): a disorder that a child develops six months after a significant death, in which unrelenting grief and sadness hasn't improved with time.

adjustment disorder with depressed mood (ADDM): a subtype of depression in which symptoms occur within three months of a stressful event but do not linger more than six months.

affect regulation: techniques to help manage the swings of moods.

affective disorders: alternative phrase used for **mood disorders**.

akinesia: a side effect of medication resulting in extreme restlessness, internal discomfort, and anxiety.

alexithymia: the inability to understand words and their textures.

amygdala: brain structure responsible for emotion and motivation.

anhedonia: the loss of pleasure and joy.

antidepressant discontinuation syndrome: negative experience that results from reducing the dosage of, or coming off of, antidepressant medication too quickly.

appoggiatura: a note that clashes with melody that creates an emotional response.

aromachology: the trend of creating personal scents for well-being.

aromatherapy: the practice of using aromas to promote physical and emotional well-being.

associative stigma: a social disqualification that results from one's connection to someone with mental illness. *See also* **courtesy stigma** and **stigma by association.**

atypical depression: a type of depression that shares many of the symptoms of **dysthymia** and **major depressive disorder**, but does not meet the criteria for either.

augmentation: the pharmacological approach of adding a supplemental medication to boost the effectiveness of current antidepressant medication.

basal ganglia: structure located deep within the brain that is involved with movement, thinking, and mood regulation.

biopsychiatry: the professional field that intersects biology and psychiatry to explain illness.

bipolar: moods that fluctuate between the lows of depression and the highs of mania.

bright light therapy: a holistic therapy for depression in which direct sunlight or artificial lights are used to regulate melatonin production.

catecholamines: neurotransmitter that boosts moods and regulates serotonin.

chromotherapy: the ancient practice of using color to heal.

chronic sorrow: the persistent and intensive sadness of parents who have children with severe mental illness.

chronicity: length and intensity of a depressive or manic episode.

circadian rhythm: regularity of daily rhythms, influenced by neurochemistry, light, and darkness.

comorbidity: having more than one medical or psychiatric disorder.

corrective emotional experience: an experience that enables one to correct past problems in a new and meaningful way.

cortisol: stress hormone released from the adrenal gland.

courtesy stigma: *See* **stigma by association** and **associative stigma.**

cyclothymia: chronic mood fluctuations of hypomania and depression that are present at least one year in a child.

cytokines: proteins that increase inflammation in the body.

deep brain stimulation: a neurosurgical procedure for depression that stimulates deep brain regions through implanted electrodes.

depression not otherwise specified (D-NOS): a diagnostic category in which depressive symptoms exist but do not clinically meet a recognized depressive disorder.

developmental milestones: expected stages children move through as they grow and develop.

***Diagnostic and Statistical Manual of Mental Disorders* (DSM):** a manual for diagnosis of mental disorders as classified by the American Psychiatric Association.

diathesis-stress model: a method that examines the interactions that occur between a person's biology, social environment, and unique temperament, to explain the development of a **mood disorder.**

discontinuation syndrome: *See* **antidepressant discontinuation syndrome.**

docosahexaenoic acid (DHA): an omega-3 fatty acid essential for health brain growth.

dopamine: an inhibitory **neurotransmitter** that is involved in regulating **mood.**

double depression: presence of **major depressive disorder** and **dysthymia** in a person.

drug therapy: another term often used for **pharmacotherapy.**

dysthymia: clinical depressive disorder less severe in intensity than **major depressive disorder** but longer in its duration.

electroconvulsive therapy (ECT): a medical procedure that uses electrical currents to induce a seizure; it is used to treat resistant depression.

endorphins: neurotransmitters that reduce pain and influence emotions.

epidemiology: the frequency and variation of a disorder within the population.

etiology: the cause or origin of a disorder.

gene: a unit of DNA that carries a specific genetic code.

hippocampus: brain structure involved in emotional regulation, learning, and memory.

hypomania: a less intensive form of mania.

hypothalamus: a walnut-sized structure that functions as a major relay station for communication in the brain.

International Classification of Diseases: a manual for the diagnosis of medical and psychiatric disorders as classified by the World Health Organization.

ketamine: a psychoactive substance gaining acceptance for use in **treatment-resistant depression.**

learned helplessness: a mental state in which a child learns to accept and not protest negative experiences.

limbic system: series of brain structures involving emotions, memory, awareness, and homeostasis.

mania: an elevated mood in which euphoria, impulsivity, irritability, racing thoughts, and decreased need for sleep significantly impair judgment and daily functioning.

major depressive disorder: clinical **mood disorder** involving unshakable sadness, despair, and fatigue.

medial prefrontal cortex: brain structure in the prefrontal cortex involving cognitions and emotions.

melancholia: a deep, persistent sadness.

melatonin: hormone that regulates **circadian rhythm.**

monotherapy: treatment of a disorder by a single method.

mood: a feeling or emotional state.

mood disorder: a chronic disturbance of mood that disrupts daily life.

mood swing: a cycling between highs and lows of affective states.

negative ion therapy: air cleaners that produce negative ions that relieve stress, improve concentration, and boost energy.

negative thinking style: thinking style that emphasizes negative outcomes.

neurobiological: having to do with the biological study of the nervous system and brain behavior.

neurochemical: the study of the chemical makeup of the brain and central nervous system.

neuroendocrine: the interactions between the nervous system and the hormones in the endocrine glands.

neurotransmitter: a chemical that helps communication between neurons.

opioids: natural morphine-like brain chemicals that ease pain.

orbitofrontal cortex: a brain structure associated with the processing of emotions.

oxytocin: feel-good hormone secreted by the pituitary gland.

partial hospital program: a hospital program involving daily supportive therapies after a work or school day.

pediatric depression: the categorical term that comprises infant, child, and adolescent depression.

personalized medicine: medical model emphasizing the unique genetic makeup of a person.

pharmacotherapy: a form of therapy that uses medication as a means to treat disease.

pineal gland: brain structure that functions as the body's time clock.

premenstrual dysphoric disorder (PMDD): severe occurrence of depressive symptoms prior to a menstrual cycle.

psychopharmacology: *See* **pharmacotherapy**.

recovery: experience of being symptom free for at least four months after achieving **remission**.

recurrence: another depressive episode after **recovery** has been attained.

relapse: a full return of depressive symptoms after **remission** but before **recovery**.

remission: the experience of being symptom free.

repetitive transcranial magnetic stimulation (rTMS): a noninvasive procedure that uses electromagnetic induction to treat depression.

resilience: the ability to overcome difficulties and function in a state of well-being.

response: improvement from the initial onset of illness.

risk factors: variables that increase the chance of developing mental or physical illness.

seasonal affective disorder (SAD): a subtype of **major depressive disorder** with a seasonal onset.

selective serotonin reuptake inhibitors (SSRIs): a class of antidepressants that block the reabsorption of the **neurotransmitter serotonin** in the brain.

serotonin: neurotransmitter that regulates behavioral and emotional expression.

serotonin syndrome: a toxic response arising from high levels of **serotonin**.

soft bipolar disorder: a term used to describe atypical **bipolar** II and **bipolar** spectrum disorders.

somatic complaints: physical aches and pains.

stigma: social disapproval or marginalizing of a person with mental illness.

stigma by association: a form of stigma that results from one's connection to someone with mental illness. *See also* **associative stigma** and **courtesy stigma**.

stressful live events (SLE): significant situations that press negatively on one's life experience.

subclinical: symptoms that fall just below the criteria for a clinical disorder.

suicidality: a range of self-harm and suicidal behaviors.

talk therapy: a term used to describe psychotherapy.

temperament: a biologically based inclination to behave in a particular way.

transcranial direct current stimulation (tDCS): an experimental, noninvasive, more refined form of ECT.

treatment-resistant depression (TRD): depression that does not respond well to traditional therapies and medications.

triggers: feelings, thoughts, or experiences that cause trauma.

unipolar: moods that are rooted in a depressive state.

vagus nerve stimulation: an implanted pacemaker that sends electrical impulses through the vagus nerve to treat depression.

vulnerability model: a model describing a child's predisposed vulnerabilities that sets the stage for illness.

well-being: the physical and emotional state of feeling content and happy.

Bibliography

ABCNews. "One in Forty Infants Experience Baby Blues, Doctors Say." ABCNews.com. Retrieved January 25, 2013, from http://abcnews.go.com/Health/OnCall/story?id=2640591&page=1.

Adams, Denise, et al. "The Safety of Pediatric Acupuncture: A Systematic Review." *Pediatrics* 128 (2011): 1011–91.

Akiskal, Hagop. "Dysthymia and Cyclothymia in Psychiatric Practice a Century after Kraepelin." *Journal of Affective Disorders* 62 (2001): 17–31.

Albert, G. C., et al. "Deep Brain Stimulation, Vagal Nerve Stimulation, and Transcranial Stimulation: An Overview of Stimulation Parameters and Neurotransmitter Release." *Neuroscience & Biobehavioral Reviews* 37 (2009): 1042–60.

American Psychiatric Association. *Diagnostic and Statistical Manual of Mental Disorders*, 5th edition. Washington, DC: American Psychiatric Association, 2013.

Andover, Margaret, and Brandon Gibb. "Non-Suicidal Self-Injury, Attempted Suicide and Suicidal Intent among Psychiatric Inpatients." *Psychiatry Research* 178 (2010): 101–5.

Azeemi, Samina, et al. "A Critical Analysis of Chromotherapy and Its Scientific Evolution." *Evidence-Based Complementary and Alternative Medicine* 2 (2005): 481–88.

Barrett, Peter, and Lucinda Barrett. "The Potential of Positive Places: Senses, Rain, and Spaces." *Intelligent Buildings International* 2 (2010): 46–52.

Bartels, Stephen J. "Caring for the Whole Person: Integrated Health Care for Older Adults with Severe Mental Illness and Medical Comorbidity." *Journal of the American Geriatric Society* 52 (2004): S249–57.

Bates, John. "Applications of Temperament Concepts." In *Temperament in Childhood*, edited by Geldolph Kohnstamm, Mary Rothbart, and John Bates, 321–55. New York: Wiley, 1989.

Baylor, Byrd, and Peter Parnall. *The Other Way to Listen*. New York: Simon & Schuster, 1978.

Beardslee, William R., and Tracy Gladstone. "Prevention of Childhood Depression: Recent Findings and Future Prospects." *Biological Psychiatry* 49 (2001): 1101–10.

Beck, Aaron, et al. *Manual for the Beck Depression Inventory-II*. San Antonio: Psychological Corporation, 1996.

Becker, Marshall, and Lois Maiman. "Sociobehavioral Determinants of Compliance with Health and Medical Care Recommendations." *Medical Care* 13 (1975): 10–24.

Bhatia, Shashi, and Subhash Bhatia. "Childhood and Adolescent Depression." *American Family Physician* 75 (2007): 73–80.

Birmaher, Boris, et al. "Childhood and Adolescent Depression: A Review of the Past 10 Years. Part I." *Journal of the American Academy of Child and Adolescent Psychiatry* 35 (1996): 1427–39.

Blier, Pierre, Daniel Zigman, and Jean Blier. "On the Safety and Benefits of Repeated Intravenous Injections of Ketamine for Depression." *Biological Psychiatry* 72 (2012): e11–12.

Bloch, Yuval, et al. "Repetitive Transcranial Magnetic Stimulation in the Treatment of Depression in Adolescents: An Open-Label Study." *Journal of ECT* 24 (2008): 156–59.

Bodnar, Richard J. "Neuropharmacological and Neuroendocrine Substrates of Stress-Induced Analgesia." *Annals of the New York Academy of Science* 467 (1986): 345–60.

Bowen-Irish, Tere. "Bringing Yoga into the Classroom: You'll Be Surprised at What It Does." *YogaKids International Articles* (2005): 418.

Boyajian, Paula. "Yoga for the Child with Special Needs." *Exceptional Parent* 4 (2004): 28–30.

Bratton, Sue, et al. "The Efficacy of Play Therapy with Children: A Meta-Analytic Review of Treatment Outcomes." *Professional Psychology: Research and Practice* 36 (2005): 376–90.

Bridge, Jeffrey A. "Clinical Response and Risk for Reported Suicidal Ideation and Suicide Attempts in Pediatric Antidepressant Treatment: A Meta-Analysis of Randomized Controlled Trials." *Journal of the American Medical Association* 297 (2007): 1683–96.

Briere, John. *Trauma Symptom Checklist for Young Children: Professional Manual.* Odessa: Psychological Assessment Resources, 2005.

Brunoni, Andre, et al. "The Sertraline vs. Electrical Current Therapy for Treating Depression Clinical Study." *JAMA Psychiatry* 1 (2013): 1–9.

"Building the Legacy." IDEA Government. Retrieved November 13, 2012, from http://idea.ed.gov.

Byrne, Peter. "Stigma of Mental Illness and Ways of Diminishing It." *Advances in Psychiatric Treatment* 6 (2000): 65–72.

Carlson, Gabrielle. "The Challenge of Diagnosing Depression in Childhood and Adolescence." *Journal of Affective Disorders* 61 (2003): 3–8.

Cash, Ralph E. "When It Hurts to Be a Teenager." *Principal Leadership Magazine* 4 (2003): 1–6.

Centers for Disease Control and Prevention. "CDC Wonder Database: Mortality Query." Centers for Disease Control. Retrieved February 17, 2013, from http://wonder.cdc.gov.

Centers for Disease Control and Prevention. "Youth Suicide and Attempted Suicide." *Morbidity and Mortality Weekly Report* 53 (2004): 471.

Cole, David, et al. "A Longitudinal Study of Cognitive Risks for Depressive Symptoms in Children and Young Adolescents." *Journal of Early Adolescence* 31 (2012): 782–16.

Compas, Bruce, Jennifer Connor-Smith, and S. S. Jaser. "Temperament, Stress Reactivity, and Coping: Implications for Depression in Childhood and Adolescence." *Journal of Clinical Child and Adolescent Psychology* 33 (2004): 21–31.

Conners, Keith. *Conners Comprehensive Behavior Rating Scales.* Austin: Pro-Ed, 2008.

Corrigan, Patrick, et al. "Stigmatizing Attitudes about Mental Illness and Allocation of Resources to Mental Health Services." *Community Mental Health Journal* 40 (2004): 297–307.

Corrigan, Patrick, and F. Miller. "Shame, Blame, and Contamination: A Review of the Impact of Mental Illness Stigma on Family Members." *Journal of Mental Health* 13 (2004): 537–48.

Corrigan, Patrick, and Amy Watson. "The Paradox of Self-Stigma and Mental Illness." *Clinical Psychology: Science and Practice* 9 (2002): 35–53.

Curry, John, et al. "Recovery and Recurrence Following Treatment for Adolescent Major Depression." *Archives of General Psychiatry* 68 (2011): 263–69.

Dalgleish, Tim, et al. "Method-of-Loci as a Mnemonic Device to Facilitate Access to Self-Affirming Personal Memories for Individuals with Depression." *Clinical Psychological Science* (2013), in press.

Darlington, Yvonne, and Robert Bland. "Strategies for Encouraging and Maintaining Hope among People Living with Serious Mental Illness." *Australian Social Work* 52 (1999): 17–24.

Davidson, Lucy, and Markku Linnoila. *Risk Factors for Youth Suicide.* New York: Taylor & Francis Group, 1990.

Dean, Carolyn. *The Miracle of Magnesium.* New York: Ballantine, 2006.

DeGangi, Georgia, et al. *Infant/Toddler Symptom Checklist: A Screening Tool for Parents.* San Antonio: Psychological Corporation, 1995.

Delate, Thomas, et al. "Trends in the Use of Antidepressants in a National Sample of Uninsured Pediatric Patients, 1988–2002." *Psychiatric Services* 55 (2004): 387–91.

Diener, Ed. "Subjective Well-Being: The Science of Happiness and a Proposal for a National Index." *American Psychologist* 55 (2000): 34–43.

Dieter, Pamela J., et al. "Self-Injury and Self-Capacities: Assisting an Individual in Crisis." *Journal of Clinical Psychology* 56 (2000): 1173–91.

Dowds, James, and Diane Stafford. *The Vitamin D Cure*. Hoboken, NJ: John Wiley & Sons, 2012.

Drevets, Wayne. "Orbitofrontal Cortex Function and Structure of Depression." *Annals of the New York Academy of Sciences* 1121 (2007): 499–527.

Egger, Helen, and Robert Emde. "Developmentally Sensitive Diagnostic Criteria for Mental Health Disorders in Early Childhood." *American Psychologist* 66 (2011): 95–106.

Elbaum, Deborah. "Special Needs Care for Adult Children: Care Options." Care .com. Retrieved March 1, 2013, from http://www.care.com/special-needs-care-options-p1145-q5906.html.

Faste, Julie, and John Preston. *Taking Charge of Bipolar Disorder*. New York: Hachette Group, 2006.

Field, Tiffany. "Exercise Research on Children and Adolescents." *Complementary Therapies in Clinical Practice* 18 (2000): 54–59.

Galantino, Mary Lou, Robyn Galbavy, and Lauren Quinn. "Therapeutic Effects of Yoga for Children: A Systematic Review of the Literature." *Pediatric Physical Therapy* 20 (2008): 66–80.

Gallagher, Kathleen. "Does Child Temperament Moderate the Influence of Parenting on Adjustment?" *Developmental Review* 22 (2002): 623–43.

Garcia-Toro, Mauro, and Iratxe Aguirre. "Biopsychosocial Model in Depression Revisited." *Medical Hypotheses* 68 (2007): 683–91.

Garstein, Maria, Samuel Putnam, and Mary Rothbart. "Etiology of Preschool Behavior Problems: Contributions of Temperament Attributes in Early Childhood." *Clinical Child and Adolescent Psychology* 33 (2004): 21–31.

Ghaziuddin, Neer, et al. "Practice Parameter for Use of Electroconvulsive Therapy with Adolescents." *Journal of the American Academy of Child and Adolescent Psychiatry* 43 (2004): 1521–39.

Gillen, Lynea, and James Gillen. *Yoga Calm for Children: Educating Heart, Mind, and Body.* Portland: Three Pebbles Press, 2007.

Gillman, P. K. "Serotonin Syndrome: History and Risks." *Fundamental and Clinical Pharmacology* 12 (2009): 482–91.

Gilman, S. E., et al. "Socio-Economic Status, Family Disruption, and Residential Stability in Childhood: Relation to Onset, Recurrence, and Remission of Major Depression." *Psychological Medicine* 33 (2003): 1341–55.

Goffman, E. *Stigma: Notes on the Management of Spoiled Identity.* Englewood, NJ: Prentice-Hall, 1963.

Goldstein, Tina, et al. "Dialectical Behavior Therapy for Adolescents with Bipolar Disorder: A 1-Year Open Trial." *Journal of the American Academy of Child and Adolescent Psychiatry* 46 (2007): 820–30.

Gómez-Pinilla, Fernando. "Brain Foods: The Effects of Nutrients on Brain Functioning." *Nature Reviews Neuroscience* 9 (2008): 568–78.

Goodman, Sheryl, and Ian Gotlib. "Risk for Psychopathology in Children of Depressed Mothers: A Developmental Model for Understanding Mechanisms of Transmission." *Psychological Review* 106 (1999): 458–90.

Gotlib, Ian, and Constance Hammen. *Handbook of Depression.* New York: Guilford Press, 2009.

Gould, Madelyn, et al. "Youth Suicide Risk and Preventive Interventions: A Review of the Past 10 Years." *Journal of the American Academy of Child and Adolescent Psychiatry* 42 (2003): 386–405.

Greenspan, Stanley, and Serena Weider. *Infant and Early Childhood Mental Health: A Comprehensive Developmental Approach to Assessment.* Arlington: American Psychiatric Association, 2005.

Gries, Lydia. "Adjustment Disorder Related to Bereavement." *Journal for Nurse Practitioners* 8 (2012): 186–94.

Harmer, Catherine, et al. "Negative Ion Treatment Increases Positive Emotional Processing in Seasonal Affective Disorder." *Psychological Medicine* 42 (2011): 1605–12.

Hawkins, J. David, et al. "Preventing Adolescent Health-Risk Behaviors by Strengthening Protection during Childhood." *Archives of Pediatric and Adolescent Medicine* 153 (1999): 226–34.

Hibbeln, Joseph. "Fish Consumption and Major Depression." *Lancet* 351 (1998): 1213.

Hill, Karen L. "Promoting Exercise Compliance: A Cognitive-Behavioral Approach." *Women and Therapy* 25 (2002): 75–90.

Högberg, Goren, et al. "Depressed Adolescents in a Case-Series Were Low in Vitamin D and Depression Was Ameliorated by Vitamin D Supplementation." *Acta Paediatrica* 101 (2012): 779–83.

Holdford, Patrick. "Depression: The Nutrition Connection." *Primary Care Mental Health* 1 (2003): 9–16.

Horn, Hildegard, et al. "Efficacy of Psychodynamic Short-Term Psychotherapy for Children and Adolescents with Depression." *Praxis der Kinderpsychologie & Kinderpsychiatrie* 54 (2005): 578–97.

Hornick, Betsy, and Roberta Larson Duyff. *American Dietetic Association: Complete Food and Nutrition Guide.* Hoboken, NJ: John Wiley & Sons, 2012.

Howard, Pierce. *The Owner's Manual for the Brain: Everyday Applications from Mind-Brain Research.* Austin: Bard Press, 2006.

Insel, Thomas, and Larry Young. "The Neurobiology of Attachment." *National Review of Neuroscience* 2 (2001): 129–36.

Jackson, Stanley. *Melancholia and Depression: From Hippocratic Times to Modern Times.* New Haven, CT: Yale University Press, 1990.

Jacobson, Colleen, and Madelyn Gould. "The Epidemiology and Phenomenology of Non-Suicidal Self-Injurious Behavior among Adolescents: A Critical Review of the Literature." *Archives of Suicide Research* 11 (2007): 129–47.

Jarski, Rosemarie. *Words from the Wise: Over 6,000 of the Smartest Things Ever Said.* New York: Skyhorse Publishing, 2007.

Juslin, Patrik N., and John Sloboda. *Handbook of Music and Emotion: Theory, Research, and Applications.* New York: Oxford University Press, 2011.

Kabat-Zinn, Jon. *Coming to Our Senses: Healing Ourselves and the World through Mindfulness.* New York: Hyperion, 2011.

Kaplan, Stephen. "The Restorative Benefits of Nature: Toward an Integrative Framework." *Journal of Environmental Psychology* 15 (1995): 169–82.

Kaplow, Julie, et al. "DSM-V Diagnostic Criteria for Bereavement-Related Disorders in Children and Adolescents: Developmental Considerations." *Psychiatry* 75 (2012): 243–66.

Kasch, Karen, et al. "Behavioral Activation and Inhibition Systems and the Severity and Course of Depression." *Journal of Abnormal Psychology* 111 (2002): 589–97.

Kashani, Jarad, et al. "Developmental Perspectives in Child and Adolescent Depressive Symptoms in a Community Sample." *American Journal of Psychiatry* 146 (1989): 871–75.

Kaslow, Nadine, et al. "Family Based Interventions for Child and Adolescent Disorders." *Journal of Marital and Family Therapy* 38 (2012): 82–100.

Kemper, Kathi, Sunita Vohra, and Richard Walls. "The Use of Complementary and Alternative Medicine in Pediatrics." *Pediatrics* 122 (2008): 1374–86.

Kim, Yong-Ku, et al. "Differences in Cytokines Between Non-Suicidal Patients and Suicidal Patients in Major Depression." *Progress in Neuro-Psychopharmacology and Biological Psychiatry* 15 (2008): 356–61.

Kindlon, Dan. *Too Much of a Good Thing: Raising Children of Character in an Indulgent Age.* New York: Miramax Books, 2001.

Kistner, Janet, et al. "Helplessness in Early Childhood: Prediction of Symptoms Associated with Depression and Negative Self-Worth." *Merrill-Palmer Quarterly* 47 (2001): 336–41.

Koplewicz, Harold. *More Than Moody: Recognizing and Treating Adolescent Depression.* New York: GP Putnam, 2003.

Kovacs, Maria. *The Children's Depression Inventory*. North Tonawanda, NY: Multi-Health Systems, 1992.

Kovacs, Maria, et al. "Childhood-Onset Dysthymic Disorder. Clinical Features and Prospective Naturalistic Outcome." *Archives of General Psychiatry* 51 (1994): 365–74.

Lasky, Tamar, et al. "Children's Hospitalizations with a Mood Disorder Diagnosis in General Hospitals in the United States 2000–2006." *Child and Adolescent Psychiatry and Mental Health* 5 (2011): 27–36.

Lawson, Andrea, and Gregory Fouts. "Mental Illness in Disney Animated Films." *Canadian Journal of Psychiatry* 49 (2004): 310–14.

Lazaratou, Helen, et al. "Parental Attitudes and Opinions on the Use of Psychotropic Medication in Mental Disorders of Childhood." *Annals of General Psychiatry* 6 (2007): 1–7.

LeClaire, Anne. *Listening Below the Noise: The Transformational Power of Silence*. New York: Harper Perennial, 2010.

Lee, Yu Jin, et al. "Direct and Indirect Effects of the Temperament and Character on Alexithymia: A Pathway Analysis with Mood and Anxiety." *Comprehensive Psychiatry* 51 (2010): 201–6.

Lenze, Shannon, Jennifer Pautsch, and Joan Luby. "Parent-Child Interaction Therapy Emotion Development: A Novel Treatment for Depression in Preschool Children." *Depression and Anxiety* 28 (2011): 153–59.

Leo, Raphael, and Jesus Salvador Ligot. "A Systematic Review of Randomized Controlled Trials of Acupuncture in the Treatment of Depression." *Journal of Affective Disorders* 97 (2007): 13–22.

Lesko, Lawrence. "Personalized Medicine: Elusive Dream or Imminent Reality?" *Clinical Pharmacology & Therapeutics* 81 (2005): 807–16.

Levenkron, Steven. *Cutting: Understanding and Overcoming Self-Mutilation*. New York: W. W. Norton, 1999.

Leyse-Wallace, Ruth. *Linking Nutrition to Mental Health*. New York: iUniverse, 2008.

Luby, Joan, et al. "The Clinical Picture of Depression in Preschool Children." *Journal of the American Academy of Child and Adolescent Psychiatry* 42 (2003): 340–48.

——. "The Clinical Significance of Preschool Depression: Impairment in Functioning and Clinical Markers of the Disorder." *Journal of Affective Disorders* 112 (2009): 111–19.

——. "Preschool Major Depressive Disorder: Preliminary Validation for Developmentally Modified DSM-IV Criteria." *Journal of the American Academy of Child and Adolescent Psychiatry* 41 (2002): 928–37.

Maalouf, Fadi, Mia Atwi, and David Brent. "Treatment-Resistant Depression in Adolescents: Review and Updates on Clinical Management." *Depression and Anxiety* 28 (2011): 946–54.

MacDonald, Kai, and Tina Marie MacDonald. "The Peptide That Binds: A Systematic Review of Oxytocin and Its Prosocial Effects in Humans." *Harvard Review of Psychiatry* 18 (2012): 39–52.

MacGregor, Peggy. "Grief: The Unrecognized Parental Response to Mental Illness in a Child." *Social Work* 39 (1994): 160–66.

Marneros, Andreas, and Frederick Goodwin. *Bipolar Disorders: Mixed States, Rapid Cycling, and Atypical Forms.* New York: Cambridge University Press, 2005.

Martin, J. K. "The Construction of Fear: Americans' Preferences for Social Distance from Children and Adolescents with Mental Health Problems." *Journal of Health and Social Behavior* 48 (2007): 50–67.

Mass, Jolanda, et al. "Morbidity Is Related to a Green Living Environment." *Journal of Epidemiology and Community Health* 63 (2009): 967–73.

McKie, Robin. "Mood Lighting Used to Boost Academic Performance at Surrey School." *The Guardian,* April 30, 2011. Retrieved on November 15, 2012, from http://www.guardian.co.uk/education/2011/may/01/mood-lighting-boost-academic-performance.

Melhem, Nadine, et al. "Phenomenology and Correlates of Complicated Grief in Children and Adolescents." *Journal of the American Academy of Child and Adolescent Psychiatry* 46 (2007): 493–99.

Mendenhall, Amy, and Katherine Mount. "Parents of Children with Mental Illness: Exploring the Caregiver Experience and Caregiver-Focused Interventions." *Families in Society* 92 (2010): 183–90.

Merikangas, Kathleen, et al. "The National Comorbidity Survey Adolescent Supplement (NCS-A): I. Background and Measures." *Journal of the American Academy of Child and Adolescent Psychiatry* 48 (2009): 367–69.

Merriam Webster. *Merriam Webster's Collegiate Dictionary*. Springfield: Merriam Webster Publishing, 2001.

Milani, Anna, Marissa Lorusso, and Massimo Molteni. "The Effects of Audiobooks on the Psychosocial Adjustment of Pre-Adolescents and Adolescents with Dyslexia." *Dyslexia* 16 (2010): 87–97.

Miller, Gregory, and Steve Cole. "Clustering of Depression and Inflammation in Adolescents Previously Exposed to Childhood Adversity." *Biological Psychiatry* 72 (2012): 34–40.

Miller, Jeffrey. *The Childhood Depression Sourcebook*. New York: McGraw Hill, 1999.

Millon, Theodore, and Carrie Millon. *Manual for the Millon Adolescent Clinical Inventory*. Minneapolis: National Computer Systems, 2006.

Milne, A. A., and Ernest Shepard. *Winnie-the-Pooh*. New York: Dutton, 1988.

Mosten, Forrest S. *Collaborative Divorce Handbook*. San Francisco: John Wiley & Sons, 2009.

Nabkasorn, Chanudda, et al. "Effects of Physical Exercise on Depression, Neuroendocrine Stress Hormones, and Physiological Fitness in Adolescent Females with Depressive Symptoms." *European Journal of Public Health* 16 (2006): 179–84.

Narrow, William E., et al. "Mental Health Service Use by Americans with Severe Mental Illnesses." *Social Psychiatry and Psychiatric Epidemiology* 35 (2000): 147–55.

National Alliance on Mental Illness. *A Family Guide: What Families Need to Know About Adolescent Depression*. Arlington: National Alliance on Mental Illness, 2011.

National Institute of Mental Health. "Antidepressant Medications for Children and Adolescents: Information for Parents and Caregivers." National Institute of Mental Health. Retrieved December 13, 2013, from http://www.nimh.nih.gov/health/topics/child-and-adolescent-mental-health/antidepressant-medications-for-children-and-adolescents-information-for-parents-and-caregivers.shtml.

National Institute of Mental Health. "Major Depressive Disorder in Children." National Institute of Mental Health. Retrieved on January 31, 2013, from http://www.nimh.nih.gov/statistics/1mdd_child.shtml.

National Marriage Project. "The Date Night Opportunity." National Marriage Project. Retrieved February 20, 2013, from http://nationalmarriageproject.org.

Nemets, Hanah, et al. "Omega-3 Treatment of Childhood Depression: A Controlled, Double-Blind Pilot Study." *American Journal of Psychiatry* 163 (2006): 1098–1100.

Nigg, Joel. "Temperament and Developmental Psychopathology." *Journal of Child Psychology and Psychiatric and Allied Disciplines* 47 (2006): 395–422.

Office of Dietary Supplements, National Institutes of Health. "Strengthening Knowledge ad Understanding of Dietary Supplements." 2005. Retrieved November 14, 2012, from http://ods.od.nih.gov.

Olshansky, Simon. "Chronic Sorrow: A Response to Having a Mentally Defective Child." *Social Casework* 43 (1962): 190–93.

Parry-Jones, William. "History of Child and Adolescent Psychiatry." In *Child and Adolescent Psychiatry: Modern Approaches*, edited by Michael Rutter, Lionel Hersov, and Eric Taylor, 794–812. Oxford: Blackwell Scientific, 1993.

Perlick, Deborah A. "Stigma as a Barrier to Recovery: Adverse Effects of Perceived Stigma on Social Adaptation of Persons Diagnosed with Bipolar Disorder." *Psychiatric Services* 52 (2001): 1627–31.

Perna, Giampaolo, Danila di Pasquale, et al. "Temperament, Character, and Anxiety Sensitivity in Panic Disorder: A High Risk Study." *Psychopathology* 45 (2012): 300–304.

Posner, Kelly, et al. "Columbia Classification Algorithm of Suicide Assessment: Classification of Suicidal Events in the FDA's Pediatric Suicidal Risk Analysis of Antidepressants." *American Journal of Psychiatry* 164 (2007): 1035–43.

Power, Mick. *Mood Disorders: A Handbook of Science and Practice*. London: John Wiley & Sons, 2004.

Price, Jonathan, et al. "Emotional Side-Effects of Selective Serotonin Reuptake Inhibitors: Qualitative Study." *British Journal of Psychiatry* 195 (2009): 211–17.

Radden, Jennifer. *The Nature of Melancholy: From Aristotle to Kristeva*. New York: Oxford University Press, 2002.

Reynolds, William. *Reynolds Adolescent Depression Scale, 2nd Edition: Short Form*. Lutz, FL: Psychological Assessment Resources, 2008.

———. *Reynolds Child Depression Scale–2*. Lutz, FL: Psychological Assessment Resources, 2010.

Rice-Evans, Catherine, and Lester Packer. *Flavonoids in Health and Disease*. New York: Marcel Dekker, 2003.

Richards, C. Steven, and Michael G. Perri. *Relapse Prevention for Depression*. Washington, DC: American Psychological Association, 2010.

Robison, Julie, et al. "A Broader View of Family Caregiving: Effects of Caregiving and Caregiver Conditions on Depressive Symptoms, Health, Work, and Social Isolation." *Psychological Science* 64 (2009): 788–98.

Rosenthal, Norman. *Winter Blues: Everything You Need to Know to Beat Seasonal Affective Disorder*, revised edition. New York: Guilford Press, 2005.

Rothbart, Mary, David E. Evans, and Stephan A. Ahadi. "Temperament and Personality: Origins and Outcomes." *Journal of Personality and Social Psychology* 78, no. 1 (2000): 122–35.

Rudd, M. David, et al. "Warning Signs for Suicide: Theory, Research, and Clinical Applications." *Suicide and Life-Threatening Behavior* 36 (2006): 255–62.

Salamon, Elliott, et al. "Sound Therapy Induced Relaxation: Down Regulating Stress Processes and Pathologies." *Medical Science Monitor* 9 (2003): RA96–RA101.

Sartorius, Norman, and Hugh Schulze. *Reducing the Stigma of Mental Illness: A Report from a Global Association*. London: Cambridge University Press, 2005.

Saylor, Conway, et al. "The Pediatric Emotional Distress Scale: A Brief
Screening Measure for Young Children Exposed to Traumatic Events."
Journal of Clinical Child Psychology 28 (1999): 70–81.

Schaefer, Charles. *Foundations of Play Therapy*. New York: John Wiley & Sons,
2011.

Schaller, Mark, et al. *Evolution, Culture, and the Human Mind*. New York:
Psychology Press, 2010.

Serani, Deborah. *Living with Depression*. Lanham, MD: Rowman & Littlefield,
2011.

Shaw, Kelly, Jane Turner, and Chris Del Mar. "Tryptophan and
5-Hydroxytryptophan for Depression." *Cochrane Database of Systematic
Reviews* 4 (2003): Cd003198.

Shonkoff, Jack, and Deborah Phillips. *From Neurons to Neighborhoods:
The Science of Early Childhood Development*. Washington, DC: National
Academies Press, 2000.

Shuman, Amy, and Jeremy P. Shapiro. "The Effects of Preparing Parents
for Child Psychotherapy on Accuracy of Expectations and Treatment
Attendance." *Community Mental Health Journal* 38 (2002): 3–16.

Sinclair, Marybetts. *Pediatric Massage Therapy*. Philadelphia: Lippincott,
Williams & Wilkins, 2004.

Sloboda, John. "Empirical Studies of Emotional Response to Music." In *Cognitive
Bases of Musical Communication*, edited by Mari Riess Jones and Susan
Holleran, 33–46. Washington, DC: American Psychological Association, 1991.

———. *Exploring the Musical Mind: Cognition, Emotions, Ability, Function*. New
York: Oxford University Press, 2005.

Smith, Shawn. *The User's Guide to the Human Mind: Why Our Brains Make Us
Unhappy, Anxious, and Neurotic and What We Can Do About It*. Oakland:
New Harbinger Publications, 2011.

Sousa, David. *How the Brain Learns*. Thousand Oaks, CA: Sage Publications,
2006.

Stein, Daniel, David Kupfer, and Alan Schatzberg. *Textbook of Mood Disorders*. Arlington: American Psychiatric Association, 2003.

Stevens, Jack, et al. "Parental Attitudes toward Children's Use of Antidepressants and Psychotherapy." *Journal of Child and Adolescent Psychopharmacology* 19 (2009): 289–96.

Substance Abuse and Mental Health Services Administration. "Depression Rates Triple between the Ages of 12 and 15 Among Adolescent Girls." July 24, 2012. Retrieved April 10, 2013, from http://www.samhsa.gov/newsroom/advisories/1207241656.aspx.

Synnott, Anthony. "Roses, Coffee, and Lovers: The Meanings of Smell." *Compendium of Olfactory Research* 19 (1994): 117–28.

Target News Service. "Depression Rates Triple between the Ages of 12 and 15 among Adolescent Girls." Health Reference Center Academic, July 25, 2012.

Terman, Michael, and Jiuan Su Terman. "Treatment of Seasonal Affective Disorder with a High-Output Negative Ionizer." *Journal of Alternative and Complementary Medicine* 1 (1995): 87–92.

Thomas, Alexander, Stella Chess, and H. G. Birch. *Temperament and Behavior Disorders in Children*. New York: New York University Press, 1968.

Thompson, Miles, and Jeremy Gauntlett-Gilbert. "Mindfulness with Children and Adolescents: Effective Clinical Application." *Clinical Child Psychology & Psychiatry* 13 (2008): 395–407.

Thompson, Renee, and Howard Berenbaum. "Shame Reactions to Everyday Dilemmas Are Associated with Depressive Disorder." *Cognitive Therapy and Research* 30 (2006): 415–25.

Turner, Heather A., and Paul A. Muller. "Long-Term Effects of Child Corporal Punishment on Depressive Symptoms in Young Adults: Potential Moderators and Mediators." *Journal of Family Issues* 25 (2004): 761–82.

U.S. Preventive Services Task Force. "Screening and Treatment for Major Depressive Disorder in Children and Adolescents: U.S. Preventive Services Task Force Recommendation Statement." *Pediatrics* 123 (2009): 1223–28.

———. "Screening for Suicide Risk: Recommendation and Rationale." *Annals of Internal Medicine* 140 (2004): 820–21.

Vant Veer-Tazelaar, Petronella, et al. "Stepped-Care Prevention of Anxiety and Depression in Late Life: A Randomized Controlled Trial." *Archives of General Psychiatry* 66 (2009): 297–304.

Verduyn, Chrissie, Julia Rogers, and Alison Wood. *Depression: Cognitive Behavioral Therapy with Children and Young People*. London: Routledge, 2009.

Villalba, Rendueles, and Colin J. Harrington. "Repetitive Self-Injurious Behavior: A Neuropsychiatric Perspective and Review of Pharmacologic Treatments." *Seminars in Clinical Neuropsychiatry* 5 (2000): 215–26.

Wahl, Otto. *Media Madness: Public Images of Mental Illness*. New Brunswick, NJ: Rutgers University Press, 1995.

Walsh, Mitzi. *Bipolar Disorders: A Guide to Helping Children and Adolescents*. Sebastopol: O'Reilly and Associates, 2000.

Wasow, Mona. *The Skipping Stone: The Rippling Effect of Mental Illness in the Family*. Palo Alto, CA: Science and Behavior Books, 1995.

White, Judith. *Aromatherapy for Men*. Bloomington: Balboa Press, 2011.

White Kress, Victoria E. "Self-Injurious Behaviors: Assessment and Diagnosis." *Journal of Counseling and Development* 81 (2003): 490–96.

Wicks-Nelson, Rita, and Allen Israel. *Abnormal Child and Adolescent Psychology*. Upper Saddle River, NJ: Pearson, 2009.

Wilansky-Traynor, Pamela, et al. "Cognitive Behavioural Therapy for Depressed Youth: Predictors of Attendance in a Pilot Study." *Journal of the Canadian Academy of Child and Adolescent Psychiatry* 19 (2010): 81–87.

World Health Organization. *Integrating Mental Health into Primary Care: A Global Perspective*. Geneva: World Health Organization, 2008.

———. *International Statistical Classification of Diseases and Related Health Problems*, 10th revision. Geneva: World Health Organization Press, 2004.

———. *Mental Health: New Understanding, New Hope. The World Health Report*. Geneva: World Health Organization, 2001.

Yu, Z. J., et al. "Vagus Nerve Stimulation: Can It Be Used in Adolescents or Children with Treatment Resistant Depression?" *Current Psychiatry* 10 (2008): 116–22.

Zalsman, G., et al. "Neurobiology of Depression in Children and Adolescents." *Child and Adolescent Psychiatric Clinics of North America* 15 (2006): 843–68.

Zero to Three. *Diagnostic Classification of Mental Health and Developmental Disorders of Infancy and Early Childhood*, revised edition. Washington, DC: Zero to Three Press, 2005.

Zuckerman, Miron, et al. "On the Importance of Self-Determination for Intrinsically Motivated Behavior." *Personality and Social Psychology Bulletin* 4 (1978): 443–46.

Index

About the Author

Deborah Serani is a go-to expert on the subject of depression. What makes her perspective unique is that she specializes in the treatment of depression and also personally lives with depression. Serani's interviews can be found in *ABC News*, *Newsday*, the *Chicago Tribune*, *Women's Health & Fitness*, the Associated Press, and affiliate radio station programs at CBS and NPR. Dr. Serani is a mental health expert for Dr. Oz's *ShareCare*, writes for *Psychology Today*, and helms the "Ask the Therapist" column for *Esperanza Magazine*. She has worked as a technical advisor for the television show *Law & Order: Special Victims Unit* and is the author of the award-winning book *Living with Depression* (2011).